theclinics.com

ORAL AND MAXILLOFACIAL SURGERY CLINICS
of North America

Perioperative Management of the Oral and Maxillofacial Surgery Patient, Part I

HARRY DYM, DDS
Guest Editor

RICHARD H. HAUG, DDS
Consulting Editor

February 2006 • Volume 18 • Number 1

SAUNDERS
An Imprint of Elsevier, Inc.
PHILADELPHIA   LONDON   TORONTO   MONTREAL   SYDNEY   TOKYO

W.B. SAUNDERS COMPANY
A Division of Elsevier Inc.

1600 John F. Kennedy Blvd., Suite 1800, Philadelphia, PA 19103-2899

http://www.oralmaxsurgery.theclinics.com

**ORAL AND MAXILLOFACIAL SURGERY
CLINICS OF NORTH AMERICA**
February 2006
Editor: John Vassallo

Volume 18, Number 1
ISSN 1042-3699
ISBN 1-4160-3569-9

Copyright © 2006 Elsevier Inc. All rights reserved. No part of this publication may be reproduced or transmitted in any form or by any means, electronic or mechanical, including photocopy, recording, or any information retrieval system, without written permission from the Publisher.

Single photocopies of single articles may be made for personal use as allowed by national copyright laws. Permission of the Publisher and payment of a fee is required for all other photocopying, including multiple or systematic copying, copying for advertising or promotional purposes, resale, and all forms of document delivery. Special rates are available for educational institutions that wish to make photocopies for non-profit educational classroom use. Permissions may be sought directly from Elsevier's Rights Department in Philadelphia, PA, USA: phone: (+1) 215 239 3804, fax: (+1) 215 239 3805, e-mail: healthpermissions@elsevier.com. Requests may also be completed on-line via the Elsevier homepage (http://www.elsevier.com/locate/permissions). In the USA, users may clear permissions and make payments through the Copyright Clearance Center, Inc., 222 Rosewood Drive, Danvers, MA 01923, USA; phone: (978) 750-8400, fax: (978) 750-4744, and in the UK through the Copyright Licensing Agency Rapid Clearance Service (CLARCS), 90 Tottenham Court Road, London W1P 0LP, UK; phone: (+44) 171 436 5931; fax: (+44) 171 436 3986. Other countries may have a local reprographic rights agency for payments.

Reprints. For copies of 100 or more, of articles in this publication, please contact the Commercial Reprints Department, Elsevier Inc., 360 Park Avenue South, New York, New York 10010-1710. Tel. (212) 633-3813 Fax: (212) 462-1935 email: reprints@elsevier.com

The ideas and opinions expressed in *Oral and Maxillofacial Surgery Clinics of North America* do not necessarily reflect those of the Publisher. The Publisher does not assume any responsibility for any injury and/or damage to persons or property arising out of or related to any use of the material contained in this periodical. The reader is advised to check the appropriate medical literature and the product information currently provided by the manufacturer of each drug to be administered to verify the dosage, the method and duration of administration, or contraindications. It is the responsibility of the treating physician or other health care professional, relying on independent experience and knowledge of the patient, to determine drug dosages and the best treatment for the patient. Mention of any product in this issue should not be construed as endorsement by the contributors, editors, or the Publisher of the product or manufacturers' claims.

Oral and Maxillofacial Surgery Clinics of North America (ISSN 1042-3699) is published quarterly by W.B. Saunders Company. Corporate and editorial offices: Elsevier, Inc., 1600 John F. Kennedy Blvd., Suite 1800, Philadelphia, PA 19103-2899. Accounting and circulation offices: 6277 Sea Harbor Drive, Orlando, FL 32887-4800. Periodicals postage paid at Orlando, FL 32862, and additional mailing offices. Subscription prices are $195.00 per year for US individuals, $295.00 per year for US institutions, $90.00 per year for US students and residents, $225.00 per year for Canadian individuals, $345.00 per year for Canadian institutions, $245.00 per year for international individuals, $345.00 per year for international institutions and $115.00 per year for Canadian and foreign students/residents. To receive student/resident rate, orders must be accompanied by name or affiliated institution, date of term, and the *signature* of program/residency coordinator on institution letterhead. Orders will be billed at individual rate until proof of status is received. Foreign air speed delivery is included in all *Clinics* subscription prices. All prices are subject to change without notice. POSTMASTER: Send address changes to *Oral and Maxillofacial Surgery Clinics of North America*, W.B. Saunders Company, Periodicals Fulfillment, Orlando, FL 32887-4800. **Customer Service: 1-800-654-2452 (US). From outside of the US, call 1-407-345-4000.**

Printed in the United States of America.

PERIOPERATIVE MANAGEMENT OF THE ORAL AND MAXILLOFACIAL SURGERY PATIENT, PART I

GUEST EDITOR

HARRY DYM, DDS, Chairman, Department of Oral and Maxillofacial Surgery, The Brooklyn Hospital Center, Brooklyn, New York; Clinical Professor, Columbia University, School of Dental and Oral Surgery, New York, New York, Senior Attending, Woodhull Medical Center, Brooklyn, New York

CONTRIBUTORS

JASON ALABAKOFF, DDS, Formerly Fellow, Department of Oral and Maxillofacial Surgery, University of Pennsylvania Medical Center, Philadelphia, Pennsylvania

RANA Y. ALI, MD, Senior Pulmonary Fellow, Division of Pulmonary and Critical Care Medicine, Department of Internal Medicine, The Brooklyn Hospital Center, Brooklyn, New York

RYAZ ANSARI, BSc, DDS, Private Practice, Manchester, Connecticut

STANLEY BODNER, PhD, Practicing Psychologist; Senior Adjunct Faculty, Adelphi University-University College, Department of Social Sciences, Garden City, New York

LEE CARRASCO, DMD, MD, Assistant Professor, Department of Oral and Maxillofacial Surgery, University of Pennsylvania Medical Center, Philadelphia, Pennsylvania

DESAI N. CHIRAG, DMD, Former Chief Resident, Department of Oral and Maxillofacial Surgery, The Brooklyn Hospital Center; Private Practice, Brooklyn, New York

HARRY DYM, DDS, Chairman, Department of Oral and Maxillofacial Surgery, The Brooklyn Hospital Center, Brooklyn, New York; Clinical Professor, Columbia University, School of Dental and Oral Surgery, New York, New York, Senior Attending, Woodhull Medical Center, Brooklyn, New York

JAMES C. FANG, DDS, MPH, Chief Resident, Department of Oral and Maxillofacial Surgery, The Brooklyn Hospital Center, Brooklyn, New York

TIRBOD FATTAHI, DDS, MD, FACS, Assistant Professor and Director of Residency Program, Division of Maxillofacial Surgery, University of Florida, Jacksonville, Florida

SETH FELDMAN, DDS, Geriatric Fellow, Harvard School of Dental Medicine, Boston, Massachusetts; Cambridge Health Alliance, Cambridge, Massachusetts

HELEN GIANNAKOPOULOS, DDS, MD, Assistant Professor, Department of Oral and Maxillofacial Surgery, University of Pennsylvania Medical Center, Philadelphia, Pennsylvania

RAMESH S. GULRAJANI, MD, FCCP, Associate Professor of Clinical Medicine, Cornell University, New York, New York; Chairman, Department of Medicine, and Director, Internal Medicine Residency Program, The Brooklyn Hospital Center, Brooklyn, New York

LESLIE R. HALPERN, DDS, MD, PhD, MPH, Assistant Professor, Department of Oral and Maxillofacial Surgery, Massachusetts General Hospital; Harvard School of Dental Medicine, Boston, Massachusetts

ANDRÉS F. HERRERA, DDS, Division of Oral and Maxillofacial Surgery and Dental Medicine, Loyola Stritch School of Medicine, Loyola University Medical Center, Maywood, Illinois

SUJATA NAIK-TOLANI, MD, FCCP, Clinical Assistant Professor of Medicine, Cornell University, New York, New York; Director, Medical Intensive Care Unit, The Brooklyn Hospital Center, Brooklyn, New York

ORRETT E. OGLE, DDS, Chief and Residency Program Director, Oral and Maxillofacial Surgery, Woodhull Medical and Mental Health Center, Brooklyn, New York; Associate Professor of Oral and Maxillofacial Surgery, Columbia University, New York, New York

PETER D. QUINN, DMD, MD, Professor and Chair, Oral and Maxillofacial Surgery, University of Pennsylvania Medical Center; University of Pennsylvania School of Dental Medicine, Philadelphia, Pennsylvania

M. SCOTT REMINICK, MD, Associate Chairman, Department of Internal Medicine; Chief, Division of Pulmonary and Critical Care Medicine, The Brooklyn Hospital Center; Clinical Assistant Professor, College of Medicine, State University of New York, Downstate Medical Center, Brooklyn, New York

HARRY C. SCHWARTZ, DMD, MD, FACS, Chief of Maxillofacial Surgery, Southern California Permanente Medical Group; Adjunct Professor of Oral and Maxillofacial Surgery, University of California, Los Angeles, California

VIVEK SHETTY, DDS, DrMedDent, Professor of Oral and Maxillofacial Surgery, University of California, Los Angeles, California

DIVYANG SORATHIA, MD, Pulmonary Medicine Fellow, Division of Pulmonary and Critical Care Medicine, The Brooklyn Hospital Center, Brooklyn, New York

MARK J. STEINBERG, DDS, MD, Division of Oral and Maxillofacial Surgery and Dental Medicine, Loyola Stritch School of Medicine, Loyola University Medical Center, Maywood, Illinois

CONTENTS

Preface ix
Harry Dym

Dedication xi
Harry Dym

Perioperative Laboratory and Diagnostic Testing—What is Needed and When? 1
Tirbod Fattahi

> Preoperative patient evaluation is an essential component of any surgical practice. A complete history and physical, along with appropriate diagnostic tests, are performed routinely to ensure a safe and predictable delivery of care. Oral and maxillofacial surgeons use this principle in everyday practice. Regardless of type of surgery and practice (office-based dentoalveolar surgery, orthognathic surgery, trauma, elective aesthetic surgery), oral and maxillofacial surgeons must formulate a decision-making process and a treatment plan regarding the perioperative management of patients. The anesthetic plan and the surgical plan must be assessed preoperatively.

Fluid and Electrolyte Management and Blood Product Usage 7
Helen Giannakopolous, Lee Carrasco, Jason Alabakoff, and Peter D. Quinn

> Traditionally, the majority of oral and maxillofacial surgery patients are young and healthy. With the ever-expanding scope of the specialty, however, more surgically extensive procedures increasingly are being performed on more medically complex patients. To optimize comprehensive patient care, oral and maxillofacial surgeons are obligated to possess a firm knowledge of the basic principles of fluid management and use a sound strategy for blood product usage.

Perioperative Risk Assessment in the Surgical Care of Geriatric Patients 19
Leslie R. Halpern and Seth Feldman

> Advances in surgical and anesthetic techniques, combined with sophisticated perioperative assessment, are factors that have contributed to an expanding number of older adults undergoing oral and maxillofacial surgery. Clinical competency and ability to evaluate carefully the pathophysiologic risk of comorbid disease become paramount in order to provide safe, expedient, and effective surgical care. This review article attempts to focus on the

importance of perioperative risk assessment in geriatric surgical patients. Specifically, medical workup of comorbid systemic illnesses and pharmacologic therapy are assessed in order to determine appropriate treatment strategies for successful surgical outcomes.

Perioperative Considerations in the Management of Pediatric Surgical Patients   35
Mark J. Steinberg and Andrés F. Herrera

> Pediatric anatomy and physiology differ significantly from those of adults and, therefore, require special considerations in evaluation and perioperative management. This article highlights the anatomic and physiologic differences that influence pediatric management. It also covers specific disease processes that are common in the pediatric population and that may involve special management strategies.

Postoperative Care of Oral and Maxillofacial Surgery Patients   49
Orrett E. Ogle

> The postoperative care of a surgical patient will depend on the site of the surgery, the nature of the surgery, the type of anesthesia used, and comorbidities from diseases of major organ systems. Despite these variables, certain general principles are applicable and are discussed in this article. Important aspects of the immediate postoperative phase and pain management are emphasized along with the concepts of general postoperative care.

Psychologic Considerations in the Management of Oral Surgical Patients   59
Stanley Bodner

> Entering the often-sterile milieu that characterizes most surgical and presurgical environments sets into motion, for most patients, emotional or psychologic reactions. At times, these inner stirrings may manifest in the form of outward behaviors, such as expressions of anxiety or anger or verbalizations suggestive of depression. The essential psychologic issue is that undergoing any surgery—minor, major, elective, or urgent—is far from an emotionally neutral event for typical oral surgical patients.

Fever Work-Up and Management in Postsurgical Oral and Maxillofacial Surgery Patients   73
Ryaz Ansari

> This article focuses on the etiology, diagnosis, and management of fever in postoperative oral and maxillofacial surgery patients. A list of the causes of postoperative fever can be exhaustive. This article focuses on the more common presentations relevant to oral and maxillofacial surgeons. Some rare but important causes also are discussed. To be comprehensive in covering this topic, a definition of fever and an overview of its pathophysiology are included.

Perioperative Management of Patients Who Have Pulmonary Disease   81
Rana Y. Ali and M. Scott Reminick

> The identification of risk factors and optimization of respiratory status are crucial to the successful management of patients who have pulmonary disease and are undergoing a surgical procedure. This article explores the approach to pulmonary patients, from the preoperative assessment to the intraoperative and postoperative periods. The management of specific pulmonary disorders in the perioperative period is discussed.

Prevention of Venous Thromboembolism 95

Divyang Sorathia, Sujata Naik-Tolani, and Ramesh S. Gulrajani

> Venous thromboembolism (VTE) is a preventable cause of significant morbidity and mortality in hospitalized patients, especially in the perioperative period. After identifying the risk factors, it is possible to stratify patients into groups based on their degree of risk for developing VTE. Methods available for the prevention of VTE vary in degree of intensity, efficacy, and side effects. The type of preventive measure used for each patient is based on matching the degree of risk for VTE with the intensity of prophylaxis, keeping in mind the risk-benefit ratio. This article discusses VTE prophylaxis relevant to oral and maxillofacial surgery patients.

Wound Healing and Perioperative Care 107

Vivek Shetty and Harry C. Schwartz

> Wounding or injury unleashes a tightly choreographed array of cellular, physiologic, biochemical, and molecular processes that restore the integrity and functional capacity of damaged tissue. Healing in the orofacial region usually is taken for granted, yet local and systemic factors can hinder the process of tissue restitution and set the stage for adverse outcomes. Although surgical attention focuses on local wound care, consideration of systemic factors is equally important. An understanding of the biologic underpinnings of the wound-healing continuum provides surgeons with a framework for developing the skills required to care for wounds and facilitate healing.

Nutritional Aspects of Care 115

James C. Fang, Desai N. Chirag, and Harry Dym

> Malnutrition in the oral and maxillofacial surgery patient can have critical implications in the overall well-being and prognosis of the long-term, hospitalized, ill patient. The OMS should be capable of assessing the patient's nutritional status and nutritional requirements and developing appropriate recommendations for proper nutritional management. Knowledge of the various modalities of nutritional support should be readily available to the OMS practitioner.

Index 131

FORTHCOMING ISSUES

May 2006
> **Perioperative Management of the OMS Patient, Part II**
> Harry Dym, DDS, *Guest Editor*

August 2006
> **Surgical Management of the Temporomandibular Joint**
> A. Thomas Indresano, DMD, *Guest Editor*

November 2006
> **Oral Cancer**
> Sanjay P. Reddi, BDS, MD, *Guest Editor*

PREVIOUS ISSUES

November 2005
> **Management of the Pediatric Maxillofacial Patient**
> Mark A. Egbert, DDS, and
> Bonnie L. Padwa, DMD, MD, FACS, *Guest Editors*

August 2005
> **The Role of the Oral and Maxillofacial Surgeon in Wartime, Emergencies, and Terrorist Attacks**
> David B. Powers, DMD, MD, *Guest Editor*

May 2005
> **Diagnosis and Management of Skin Cancer**
> Michael S. Goldwasser, DDS, MD, and
> Jonathan S. Bailey, DMD, MD, FACS, *Guest Editors*

THE CLINICS ARE NOW AVAILABLE ONLINE!

Access your subscription at:
www.theclinics.com

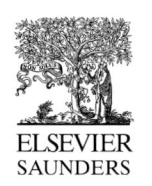

Preface

Perioperative Management of the Oral and Maxillofacial Surgery Patient, Part I

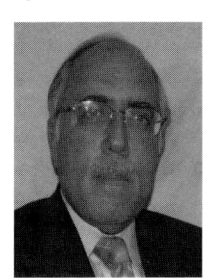

Harry Dym, DDS
Guest Editor

Like many in our esteemed profession, I have spent my entire professional life (over 28 years) working almost exclusively in a hospital setting within an American Dental Association–approved Oral and Maxillofacial Surgery Residency Training Program. Much has changed during this time, mostly for the better.

As the national percentage of older (ie, over 65 years of age) Americans continues to grow and our profession's scope of services continues to increase, it is becoming quite evident that our patient practice demographics will also begin to shift. As a profession, we will begin performing more complex reconstructive procedures on patients who have compromised health histories.

It is with that thought in mind that this two-part issue was planned: to serve as a text and reference work for better management in the perioperative care of the medically compromised and hospitalized patient segment of our practices. We hope that the readership will find this two part series useful and valuable to their everyday clinical practice.

On a personal note, being involved with the *Oral and Maxillofacial Surgery Clinics of North America* is always a most rewarding and fulfilling experience, and I would like to thank John Vassallo, Editor, for his support and assistance. To the Senior Administration of The Brooklyn Hospital Center, Mr. Sam Lehrfeld, President and Chief Executive Officer, Mr. Paul Albertson, Senior VP Operation/Ambulatory Care, Mr. Rick Braun, Executive VP/CFO, and Dr. John Carroll, Chief Medical Officer, I offer my sincere thanks for their complete and uncompromising support of the Department of Dentistry and Oral & Maxillofacial Surgery, and of our department's dual mission of quality patient care and resident education.

I have been fortunate to have spent the past quarter of a century working under and with the following three people: Dr. Peter Sherman, Chairman of Dental/OMS at Woodhull Hospital Medical Center, who has been a valued colleague and cherished friend, along with Dr. Earl Clarkson, Director of Dentistry/Oral and Maxillofacial Surgery at the Brooklyn Hospital Center, and Dr. Orrett Ogle, Chief of OMS at Woodhull, who contributed to this issue. They are true stars of our profession, and I am fortunate to have had them by my side for constant support and encouragement these many years.

Equally rewarding when editing a two-part text such as this are the oral and maxillofacial surgery colleagues I've come to know and work with. I am privileged to have had Drs. Leslie Halpern, Peter Quinn, Larry Cunningham, Ryaz Ansari, Guillermo Chacon, Mark Steinberg, Andrés Herrera, Stanley Bodner, Desai Chirag, James Fang, Scott Reminick,

Sanjeev Raj Bhatia, Ramesh Gulrajani, Hyon Yoo, Bethany Serafin, Tirbod Fattahi, Ladi Doonquah, Vivek Shetty, Harry Schwartz, Lee Carrasco, Leon Assael, and Remy H. Blanchaert, Jr., assisting me in this work. They have all successfully completed their mission, and I look forward to working with them again on future projects. Corinne Acevedo, my Executive Assistant, played a major role in coordinating the editorial material, and I thank her for her patience, diligence, and excellent work.

Finally, I must acknowledge my family for their consistent and steadfast support despite too many hours spent in the hospital and away from home: Freidy, my beautiful wife of 28 years, my oldest son Yehoshua, my daughter-in-law Chani, my other two boys, Daniel and Akiva, and my beautiful and talented daughter Hindy.

This issue is dedicated to my parents, Mollie Dym and Chaim Dym; to my mother-in-law, Hedy Rosner; and my late father-in-law, Sol Rosner, a wonderful person who is sorely missed. They all embody and represent what is noble, ethical, moral, and good and are a beacon of light that helps guide me in my journey through this life.

Harry Dym, DDS
The Brooklyn Hospital Center
121 DeKalb Avenue
Brooklyn, NY 11201, USA
E-mail address: hdymdds@yahoo.com

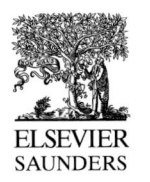

Dedication

This issue is dedicated to the memory of my mother, Molly Dym, who passed away suddenly and departed from this world on Saturday, November 19, 2005. My mother came to America as an immigrant in 1950 having survived the raging flames and inferno of Nazi Europe. She arrived on these shores poor in worldly possessions but rich in spirit and dreams of a brighter future for her and my dear father.

My mother was a devoutly religious woman who believed firmly in God, family, and education. She fought valiantly against the ravages of Parkinson's disease and died, with her family at her side, having fulfilled her dream.

Harry Dym, DDS

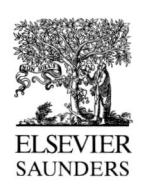

Perioperative Laboratory and Diagnostic Testing—What is Needed and When?

Tirbod Fattahi, DDS, MD, FACS

Division of Maxillofacial Surgery, University of Florida, 653-1 West 8th Street, Jacksonville, FL 32209, USA

Preoperative patient evaluation is an essential component of any surgical practice. A complete history and physical, along with appropriate diagnostic tests, are performed routinely to ensure a safe and predictable delivery of care. Oral and maxillofacial surgeons use this principle in everyday practice. Regardless of type of surgery and practice (office-based dentoalveolar surgery, orthognathic surgery, trauma, elective aesthetic surgery), oral and maxillofacial surgeons must formulate a decision-making process and a treatment plan regarding the perioperative management of patients. The anesthetic plan and the surgical plan must be assessed preoperatively.

Preoperative evaluation of surgical patients and the decisions regarding choosing the appropriate and specific presurgical laboratory tests can be a daunting task at times because often it is riddled with confusion and ambiguity. The dilemma facing healthcare providers is twofold: one, there is the need to reduce or eliminate nonindicated preoperative tests; two, there is a responsibility to continue to order indicated tests to maximize and improve patient care. There is no doubt that there exist some limitations regarding preoperative testing of surgery patients. One of the first difficulties faced by clinicians is the definition of the word, "abnormal." When ordering a test, clinicians are attempting to discriminate between patients who have normal values and those who have abnormal ones. This knowledge then is used to determine the possibility for the existence of a pathologic condition, which ultimately may have an impact on the proposed surgical and anesthetic plan. Unfortunately, most laboratory values are based on a 95% confidence limit; therefore, it is possible that 5% of "normal" patients who do have any pathologic condition have an "abnormal" test result [1]. This may lead to misinterpretation of a pathologic condition. It is just as important to consider not only if a laboratory value is abnormal but also if an abnormal value may affect the perioperative care of patients or is able to predict a complication [2]. It is estimated that only 0.22% of all "abnormal" preoperative tests done before elective surgery could influence the perioperative management of the surgical patients [3].

It is estimated that the health care industry spends 20 to 30 billion dollars annually on preoperative laboratory testing in this country [4]. This is an enormous expense considering the volume of scientifically based studies refuting the benefits of routine preoperative laboratory work. A 1-year study of outpatient surgical patients at a teaching hospital reveals the potential of more than $400,000 in cost reduction if preoperative laboratory tests had been ordered properly [2].

A PubMed search for "preoperative laboratory testing" reveals more than 200 articles. A quick review of these articles demonstrates a paucity of scientific evidence to validate the benefits of a random, preoperative testing paradigm. The American Society of Anesthesiologists (ASA) Task Force on Preanesthesia Evaluation released its report in February of 2002 [5]. The task force was unable to issue true practice standards or guidelines based on strict evidence-based information because of a lack of an adequate number of controlled scientific studies. Instead, a practice advisory report was formulated

E-mail address: Tirbod.Fattahi@jax.ufl.edu

based on noncontrolled studies, opinions of consultants, and a sample of common practices [6]. Unfortunately, this advisory report not always is enforced or used at every medical center or practice. Pasternak aptly states, "... in the past, there existed an assumption that all elective surgical procedures must be preceded by a series of comprehensive tests, regardless of the patient's age, health status, or planned procedures. The traditional system of the protocol 'battery of tests' evolved from a lack of clear definition of their role in preoperative screening, insufficient information on their utility, and a mistaken belief that voluminous information, no matter how extraneous, enhanced the safety of care and reduced physician liability for adverse events" [7]. The object of laboratory testing should be to assist in the decision-making process when planning surgical or anesthetic intervention; laboratory testing is a complement, not a substitute for, a good, accurate history and physical.

It also is imperative to note that although there are medical practices based on personal preference and anecdotal experience, there still are many irrefutable studies supporting proper preoperative evaluation for elective surgery [8–10]. One large study documents at least one complication in 17% of all surgical patients [9]. This and other studies demonstrate an overall increased risk for surgical morbidity and mortality associated with advanced age; therefore, appropriate preoperative tests are recommended based solely on the age of patients [9,10].

The purpose of this article is to provide a comprehensive review of the current literature regarding appropriate preoperative assessment of patients undergoing oral and maxillofacial surgery. Unfortunately, because of contradictory data, lack of randomized studies, and absence of a consistent system for risk assessment, the recommendations listed in this article are suggested screening tools based on specific clinical conditions. At attempt is made to include as many of the routine and useful preoperative tests as possible. Clinicians also are advised to become familiar with trends and policies of affiliated medical institutions and surgical centers, because slight variations may exist. The majority of policies regarding preoperative assessment of surgical patients are determined by the department of anesthesiology in most medical centers.

Recommended guidelines

Familiarity with the ASA patient classification is critical when performing a preoperative patient assessment (Table 1). The ASA classification is a universally accepted, overall impression of surgical patients who are to undergo an anesthetic procedure. Preoperative risk stratification also can include a surgical classification system (Table 2) [4]. This classification is especially useful for healthy patients undergoing a surgical procedure, because risk assessment is determined solely by the nature of the procedure rather than the ASA classification. Regardless of the classification system used, a complete history and physical is the most important parameter for patient assessment during the preoperative period. Preoperative testing should be ordered only for those conditions that may have an impact on the perioperative management of patients, including [4]

Table 1
American Society of Anesthesiologists Patient Classification

ASA Class I	Healthy patients
ASA Class II	Patients who have mild systemic disease
ASA Class III	Patients who have severe systemic disease that limits activity but is not incapacitating
ASA Class IV	Patients who have an incapacitating systemic disease that is a constant threat to life
ASA Class V	Moribund patients not expected to survive 24 hours with or without an operation

Note: if a surgical procedure is performed emergently, an "E" is added to the previously defined ASA classification.

- Medical status of patients (ASA classification or presence of a specific condition based on patient history and physical)
- Nature of the surgical procedure (surgical classification system)
- Nature of the anesthetic technique
- Patient inclusion in a high-risk group based on epidemiology (eg, ECG for age ≥ 40)
- Baseline determination requirements because of likely changes resulting from the surgery or postoperative interventions

Testing without specific indications is shown to be neither of clinical benefit nor cost effective [2,11–18]. Furthermore, such action may increase patient discomfort and augment the potential adverse effects of further assessment of clinically unimportant, yet ordered and documented, laboratory abnormalities.

After reviewing the current literature, certain conclusions can be derived regarding choosing appropriate preoperative laboratory tests. Figs. 1

Table 2
Surgical classification system

Category 1	Minimal risk to patients independent of anesthesia Minimally invasive procedures with little or no blood loss Often done in an office setting
Category 2	Minimal to moderately invasive procedure Blood loss less than 500 μL Mild risk to patients independent of anesthesia
Category 3	Moderately to significantly invasive procedure Blood loss potential 500–1500 μL Moderate risk to patients independent of anesthesia
Category 4	Highly invasive procedure Blood loss greater than 1500 μL Major risk to patients independent of anesthesia

and 2 and Tables 3 and 4 list current recommendations regarding appropriate preoperative patient assessment.

Several comments need to be made regarding the current recommendations. First and foremost, clinicians must realize that the recommendations are suggestions; as stated previously, there is no standardized testing paradigm. Other testing methods, in addition to the current recommendations, may be warranted based on patient clinical condition or other concomitant diseases.

Although age alone should not be an indication for preoperative tests, most healthy patients of advanced age are at increased risk for perioperative complications [9,10,19]. Specific criteria, therefore, are established to address this issue (see Table 4). It is imperative to remember that age-specific re-

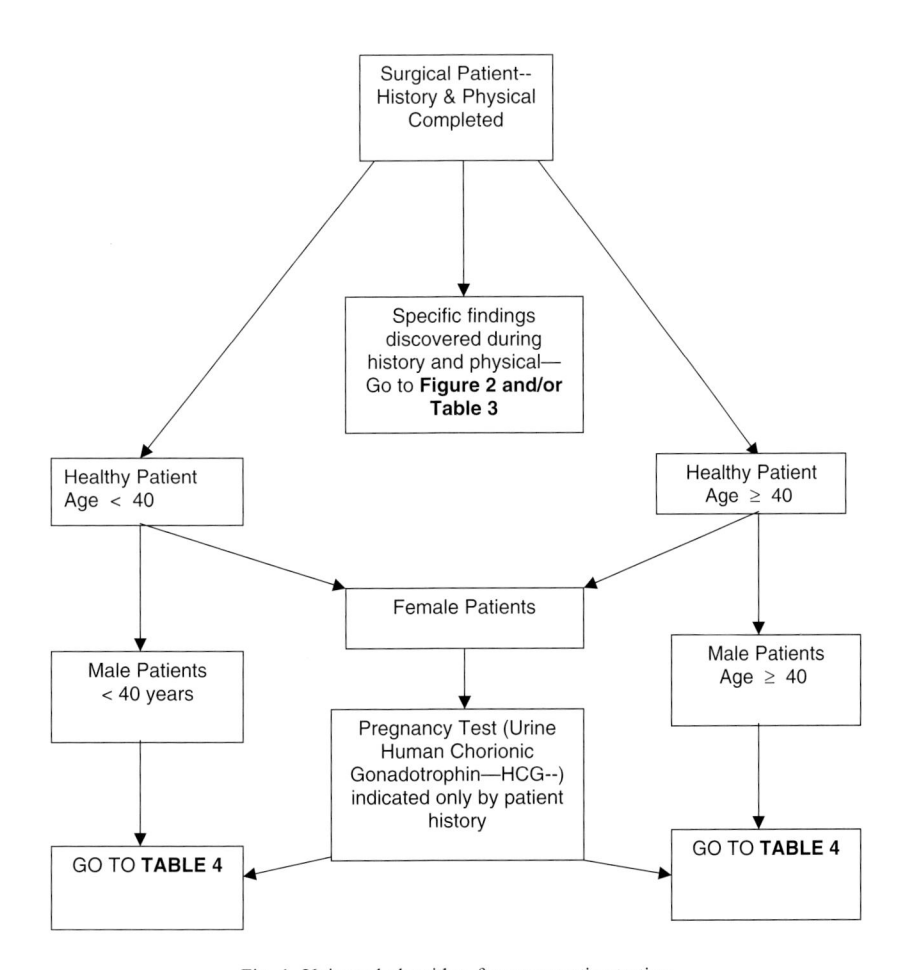

Fig. 1. Universal algorithm for preoperative testing.

```
                    ┌─────────────────────┐
                    │  Surgical Patient   │
                    │  ASA Classification │
                    │     Determined      │
                    └──────────┬──────────┘
             ┌─────────────────┴─────────────────┐
             ▼                                   ▼
       ┌──────────┐                    ┌──────────────────┐
       │  ASA I   │                    │  ASA II or Greater│
       │          │                    │   Regardless of   │
       │          │                    │ Surgical Category │
       └────┬─────┘                    └─────────┬────────┘
            │                                    ▼
            │                           ┌────────────────┐
            │                           │ Go to Table 3  │
            │                           └────────────────┘
```

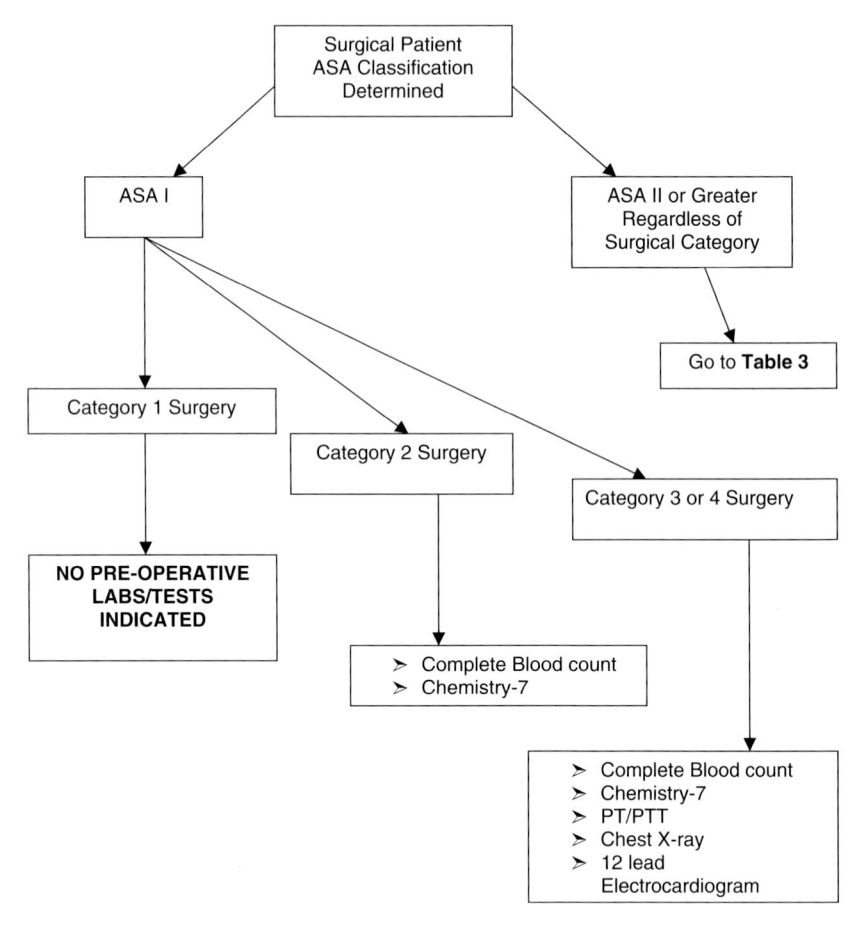

Fig. 2. Indications for routine preoperative laboratory testing based on patient ASA and surgical classification system (independent of patient age).

quirements are independent of other patient factors, such as ASA classification or nature of the planned surgical procedure. For example, a healthy 45-year-old patient undergoing an elective outpatient surgical procedure may not require as many preoperative tests as a 45-year-old patient who has a significant cardiovascular history and is undergoing the same operation.

Preoperative assessment of pediatric patients also has been evaluated. As for adult patients, many practitioners continue the practice of ordering non-indicated tests for pediatric patients. Studies show no clinical benefit of routine preoperative laboratory testing in children undergoing outpatient or noninvasive surgical procedures [20,21].

Preoperative assessment of female patients of childbearing age also is of interest. One of every 10 women between 15 and 19 years of age becomes pregnant each year in the United States and more than 95% of these pregnancies are unplanned [22]. It is conceivable, therefore, that some of these patients may present for elective surgical procedures. Although there are few data regarding the teratogenic effects of anesthetics on the developing fetus, there is a significant risk of spontaneous abortion, intrauterine growth retardation, and prematurity if a pregnant female is anesthetized during the first trimester. Based on these facts, a recent national survey reveals that 27% of all practitioners routinely order a urine pregnancy test in adolescent patients before surgery [22]. There are a number of multicenter studies indicating, however, that the potential for an unrecognized pregnancy, following a detailed history and physical with specific questions regarding the last

Table 3
Indications for commonly ordered preoperative laboratory tests based on specific findings during history and physical examination (independent of patient age, American Society of Anesthesiologists classification, or surgical procedure)

Test	Indications
Complete blood count	Recent infection
	Immune compromised states (ie, HIV)
	History of cancer
	Chemotherapy or radiation treatment
	Fever
	Corticosteroid use
	Anticoagulation medications
Hemoglobin	History of anemia
	Anticipated high blood loss
	Malignancy
	History of gastrointestinal bleed
Platelet count	Bleeding history
	Thrombopathy
	Splenectomy
	Liver disease
	Autoimmune disease
Chemistry-7	Malnutrition/dehydration
	Corticosteroid use
	Diuretic use
	Digitalis use
	Renal failure
	Diabetes
	Infection
Blood glucose	Steroid therapy
	Diabetes
	Pancreatic disease
	Adrenal disease
	Pituitary disease
Prothrombin time/partial thromboplastin time, bleeding time	Bleeding disorders
	Coagulopathy
	Jaundice
	Chronic renal failure
	Alcoholism
	Anticoagulation medications
	Liver disease
	History of stroke
	Evidence of purpura or petechiae
Liver function tests	Malnutrition
	Liver disease/hepatitis/jaundice
	Pancreatic disease
	History of cancer
	Alcoholism
	Hepatomegally
Urinalysis/urine pregnancy test	Dysuria
	Pregnancy
Chest radiograph	Cardiovascular disease
	Lung disease (obstructive and restrictive airways diseases, shortness of breath)
	Upper respiratory infections
	Chronic smoking

Table 3 (*continued*)

Test	Indications
12-lead ECG	History of cardiac disease
	Chest pains
	Lung disease
	Morbid obesity
	History of stroke
Echocardiogram	Recent myocardial infarction
	Congestive heart failure
	Abnormal ECG
	Unstable angina
	Significant arrhythmia
	Severe valvular disease

menstrual cycle, is less that 0.5% [22–24]. Routine preoperative urine human chorionic gonadotrophin testing in the female adolescent surgical population, therefore, may not be necessary.

Summary

There is no doubt that clinicians are faced with conflicting data when deciding on the appropriate preoperative tests for surgical patients. As discussed previously, the ASA, one of the major regulating bodies involved in the perioperative care of surgical patients, is unable to issue standardized testing protocols for patient assessment. This only highlights the dysfunctional and costly current practice of ordering a battery of tests before surgery for every surgical patient, regardless of age, ASA status, or findings on history and physical examination. There is no substitute for a properly performed and detailed history and physical examination. Data suggests that most clinically relevant conditions are recognized during the history and physical examination without the need for further laboratory testing [25–27]. Review of the current literature cited in this article confirms this finding. Most ASA I patients under-

Table 4
Indications for routine preoperative laboratory testing based on patient age only

Age	Indicated tests
Healthy patient under age 40	No routine preoperative tests indicated unless major blood loss or major hemodynamic changes anticipated
Healthy patient age 40 or older	Complete blood count
	12-lead ECG
	Chest radiograph

going an elective, outpatient procedure in an oral and maxillofacial surgery office do not need any preoperative testing based on current clinical data and suggestions. It is warranted, however, to restate that specific laboratory testing is indicated based on key findings during a history and physical examination. The tables cited in this article are guidelines based on current literature; variations from the suggesting testing protocol may be warranted based on patients' surgical condition or other concomitant diseases.

References

[1] Schoen I, Brooks S. Judgment based on 95% confidence limits: a statistical dilemma involving multitest screening and proficiency testing of multiple specimens. Am J Clin Pathol 1970;53:190–5.

[2] Wattsman TA, Davies RS. The utility of preoperative laboratory testing in general surgery patients for outpatient procedures. Am Surg 1997;63:81–90.

[3] Kaplan EB, Sheiner LB, Boeckman AJ, et al. The usefulness of preoperative laboratory screening. JAMA 1985;253:3576–81.

[4] Pasternak LR. Preoperative assessment: guidelines and challenges. Acta Anaesthesiol Scand Suppl 1997;111: 318–20.

[5] American Society of Anesthesiologists Task Force on Preanesthesia Evaluation. Practice advisory for preanesthesia evaluation. Anesthesiology 2002;96: 485–96.

[6] Maurer WG, Borkowski RG, Parker BM. Quality and resource utilization in managing preoperative evaluation. Anesthesiology Clin North Am 2004;22: 155–75.

[7] Pasternak LR. Preoperative laboratory testing: general issues and considerations. Anesthesiology Clin North Am 2004;22:13–25.

[8] Roizen MF. Routine preoperative evaluation. In: Anesthesia. Churchill Livingston; 1986. p. 225–53.

[9] Khuri SF, Daley J, Henderson W, et al. The National Veterans Administration Surgical Risk Study: risk adjustment for the comparative assessment of the quality of surgical care. J Am Coll Surg 1995;180:519–31.

[10] King MS. Preoperative evaluation. Am Fam Physician 2000;62:387–96.

[11] Velanovich V. Preoperative laboratory screening based on age, gender, and concomitant medical disease. Surgery 1994;115:56–61.

[12] Halaszynski TM, Juda R, Silverman DG. Optimizing postoperative outcomes with efficient preoperative assessment and management. Crit Care Med 2004; 32(Suppl):S76–86.

[13] Velanovich V. How much routine preoperative laboratory testing is enough. Am J Med Qual 1993;8: 145–51.

[14] Smetana GW, Macpherson DS. The case against routine preoperative laboratory testing. Med Clin North Am 2003;87:7–40.

[15] Wagner JD, Moore DL. Preoperative laboratory testing for the oral and maxillofacial surgery patient. J Oral Maxillofac Surg 1991;49:177–82.

[16] Fleisher LA. Preoperative cardiac evaluation. Anesthesiology Clin North Am 2004;22:59–75.

[17] Haug RH, Reifeis RL. A prospective evaluation of the value of preoperative laboratory testing for office anesthesia sedation. J Oral Maxillofac Surg 1999;57: 16–20.

[18] Narr BJ, Warner ME, Schroeder DR, et al. Outcomes of patients with no laboratory assessment before anesthesia and a surgical procedure. Mayo Clin Proc 1997;72:505–9.

[19] Dzankic S, Pastor D, Gonzales C, et al. The prevalence and predictive value of abnormal preoperative laboratory tests in elderly surgical patients. Anesth Analg 2001;93:301–8.

[20] O'Connor ME, Drasner K. Preoperative laboratory testing of children undergoing elective surgery. Anesth Analg 1990;70:176–80.

[21] Patel RI, DeWitt L, Hannallah RS. Preoperative laboratory testing in children undergoing elective surgery:analysis of current practice. J Clin Anesthesiol 1997;9:569–75.

[22] Malviya S, D'Errico C, Reynolds C, et al. Should pregnancy test be routine in adolescent patients prior to surgery? Anesth Analg 1996;83:854–8.

[23] Manley S, de Kelaita G, Joseph N, et al. Preoperative pregnancy testing in ambulatory surgery: incidence and impact of positive results. Anesthesiology 1995; 83:690–3.

[24] Pierre N, Moy LK, Redd S, et al. Evaluation of a pregnancy-testing protocol in adolescents undergoing surgery. J Pediatr Adolesc Gynecol 1998;11: 139–41.

[25] Sandler G. Cost of unnecessary tests. Br J Med 1979; 2:21–4.

[26] Bordage G. Where are the history and the physical? CMAJ 1995;1:517–8.

[27] Peterson MC, Holbrook JH, Von Hales D, et al. Contributions of the history, physical examination, and laboratory investigation in making medical diagnoses. West J Med 1992;156:163–5.

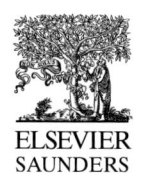

ORAL AND MAXILLOFACIAL SURGERY CLINICS of North America

Fluid and Electrolyte Management and Blood Product Usage

Helen Giannakopoulos, DDS, MD[a], Lee Carrasco, DMD, MD[a], Jason Alabakoff, DDS[a], Peter D. Quinn, DMD, MD[a,b],*

[a]Department of Oral and Maxillofacial Surgery, University of Pennsylvania Medical Center, Philadelphia, PA, USA
[b]University of Pennsylvania School of Dental Medicine, Philadelphia, PA, USA

Traditionally, the majority of oral and maxillofacial surgery patients are young and healthy. With the ever-expanding scope of the specialty, however, more surgically extensive procedures increasingly are being performed on more medically complex patients. To optimize comprehensive patient care, oral and maxillofacial surgeons are obligated to possess a firm knowledge of the basic principles of fluid management and use a sound strategy for blood product usage.

A brief review of the anatomy and composition of body fluids

Water makes up 50% to 70% of total body weight. The percentage of water is a function of multiple variables, including age and body mass. Because fat contains little water, with increasing body fat, the percentage of total body water decreases. Total body water is divided into intracellular and extracellular compartments. The extracellular compartment is subdivided into the intravascular and interstitial spaces. The intravascular space contains the plasma volume (Table 1).

* Corresponding author. Hospital of University of Pennsylvania, Department of Oral and Maxillofacial Surgery, 5th Floor, White Building, 3400 Spruce Street, Philadelphia, PA 19104.
 E-mail address: peter.quinn@uphs.upenn.edu (P.D. Quinn).

Sodium and potassium are the principal cations in the body. Sodium is contained primarily in the extracellular fluid and potassium in the intracellular fluid. Chloride is the principal anion in the body and is restricted primarily to the extracellular fluid. The electrolyte composition of body water is detailed in Table 2.

Normal exchange of fluid and electrolytes

The internal fluid environment is maintained by intimate interactions between the brain, kidneys, lungs, gastrointestinal tract, and skin. Surgical stresses that compromise any one of these systems may alter the fluid and electrolyte balance.

Under normal conditions, a 70-kg adult consumes an average of 2000 to 2500 mL of water per day [1]. Approximately 1500 mL of water is taken by mouth; the remaining water is extracted from solid food. Daily water losses include approximately 250 mL in stool, 800 to 1500 mL in urine, and 600 mL in insensible losses [1]. Insensible loss of water occurs via the skin and the lungs. Hypermetabolism, hyperventilation, and fever increase insensible water loss. With excessive heat production, insensible loss via the skin is exceeded, and sweating occurs. Insensible losses may exceed over 300 mL per day per degree of temperature above 100.5°F. Patients who have a tracheostomy have an additional risk for insensible loss. An unhumidified tracheostomy with hyperventilation may result in insensible water losses of

Table 1
Body fluid compartments

Total body water	Body weight (%)	Total body water (%)
Intracellular	40	67
Extracellular	20	33
Intravascular	5	8
Interstitial	15	25
Total	60	100

Table 3
Water exchange (70-kg man)

Route	Average daily volume (mL)	Minimal (mL)	Maximal (mL)
H_2O gain			
Sensible			
Oral fluids	800–1500	0	1500/h
Solid Foods	500–700	0	1500
Insensible			
Water of oxidation	250	125	800
Water of solution	0	0	500
H_2O loss			
Sensible			
Urine	800–1500	300	1400/h
Intestinal	0–250	0	2500/h
Sweat	0	0	4000/h
Insensible			
Lungs and skin	600	600	1500

more than 1.5 liters per day. Table 3 details routes of water exchange [1].

The goal of fluid maintenance therapy is to replace fluids lost normally during the course of a day. The standard recommendations for the calculation of hourly maintenance fluid replacement are 0 to 10 kg, 4 mL/kg; 11 to 20 kg, 2 mL/kg; and greater than 20 kg, 1 mL/kg. For example, for a 70-kg patient, $(4 \times 10) + (2 \times 10) + (1 \times 50) = 110$ mL/h. For patients weighing 20 kg or more, simply adding 40 mL to their kilogram weight allows a quicker calculation. For example, for a 70-kg patient, $70 + 40 = 110$ mL/h.

There are many electrolyte solutions available for parenteral administration. Commonly used electrolytes solutions are listed in Table 4 [2]. Selection of the appropriate fluid is determined by several factors, including patients' maintenance requirements, existing fluid deficits, and anticipated ongoing fluid losses.

For surgical patients, ongoing fluid losses are estimated and measured. Third-space losses refer to the transfer of body fluids from the extracellular space to the nonfunctional interstitial or nonintravascular spaces. Third-space losses and insensible fluid losses must be projected and replaced in addition to the calculated maintenance requirement. The correction of insensible water losses intraoperatively requires the administration of crystalloid solution at approximately 2 mL/kg/h. The recommended fluid replacement for third-space losses is outlined in Table 5. Surgeons must recognize that by 72 hours postoperatively, third-space losses become mobilized, which results in increased intravascular volume.

The quantification of intraoperative blood loss can be variable. Surgeons generally underestimate blood loss by 15% to 40%. Ongoing losses from nasogastric tubes, fistulae, and drains can be measured directly. Blood-soaked sponges may be weighed to

Table 2
Electrolyte composition of intracellular and extracellular fluid

Fluid	Plasma	Interstitial fluid	Intracellular
Cations			
Na^+	140	146	12
K^+	4	4	150
Ca^{2+}	5	3	10^{-7}
Mg^{2+}	2	1	7
Anions			
Cl^-	103	114	3
HCO_3^-	24	27	10
SO_4^{2-}	1	1	0
HPO_4^{3-}	2	2	116
Organic anions	5	5	0
Protein	16	5	40

Table 4
Electrolyte composition of commonly used intravenous solutions

Solution	Na^+	K^+	Ca^{2+}	Mg^{2+}	Cl^-	HCO_3^-
0.9% NaCl	154				154	
0.45% NaCl	77				77	
0.33 NaCl	56				56	
0.2% NaCl	34				34	
Lactated Ringer's	130	4	4		109	28
3% NaCl	513				513	
5% NaCl	855				855	

Table 5
Replacement of third-space losses

Surgeries causing	ml/kg/h
Minimal trauma	3–4
Moderate trauma	5–6
Severe trauma	7–8

estimate blood loss. One gram is equivalent to 1 mL of blood. Laparotomy sponges can hold up to 100 mL of blood. A Ray-Tec sponge holds approximately 10 to 20 mL of blood and 4 × 4 sponges hold 10 mL of blood. Suction canister volume (after subtraction of irrigation) also assists in blood loss assessment.

Body fluid disturbances can be classified into three broad categories: (1) changes in volume (hypovolemia and hypervolemia), (2) changes in concentration (hyponatremia and hypernatremia), and (3) changes in composition (acid-base imbalances and concentration changes in calcium, magnesium, and potassium). Acid-base disorders are not discussed in this article.

Intravascular fluid volume status must be assessed preoperatively. Anesthetics can cause systemic vasodilation or myocardial depression. The resultant hypotension from these effects of anesthesia can be severe in hypovolemic patients. The patient's mental status, history of recent intake and output, blood pressures, and heart rate easily are obtainable and provide important information regarding potential fluid imbalances. Several other physical signs and symptoms indicate fluid status (Box 1).

For patients in whom a fluid imbalance is suspected or patients in whom fluid imbalances are anticipated,

Box 1. Physical signs and symptoms of fluid volume imbalance

Hypovolemia	Hypervolemia
Poor skin turgor	Shortness of breath at rest or with exertion
Dry mucous membranes	JVD
Dry axilla	S3
Flat neck veins	Hepatojugular reflex
Tachycardia	Ascites
Orthostatic hypotension	Pitting edema
Hypothermia	Weight gain
Weight loss	
Sunken eyes	

Box 2. Common laboratory tests to evaluate body fluid disturbances

Hypovolemia	Hypervolemia
Serum electrolytes	Serum electrolytes
SUN/Cr	Urine-specific gravity
Hematocrit	24-hour urine for Cr clearance
Urine electrolytes and specific gravity serum albumin	Total protein
24-hour urine for Cr clearance	Cholesterol
	Liver enzymes
	Bilirubin

preoperative laboratory tests are warranted. Commonly ordered laboratory tests to evaluate fluid balance disorders are listed in Box 2. The serum urea nitrogen (SUN)/creatinine (Cr) ratio is the standard for assessing fluid status quickly.

Sodium

Normal serum sodium level is 135 to 145 mEq/L. Hyponatremia is defined as serum sodium levels less than 135 mEq/L. Acute symptomatic hyponatremia usually does not become clinically evident until serum sodium levels of 130 mEq/L. Chronic hyponatremic states usually remain asymptomatic until serum sodium levels fall below 120 mEq/L. Box 3 lists the common signs and symptoms of hyponatremia. Serum osmolality is the laboratory test most critical for the diagnosis of hyponatremia.

The first step in the management of hyponatremia is to establish the fluid volume status. The etiology

Box 3. Signs and symptoms of hyponatremia

Confusion
Lethargy
Stupor
Coma
Nausea
Vomiting
Headache
Muscle twitches
Seizures

Table 6
Etiology and management of hyponatremia

Hyponatremia	Etiology	Treatment
Iso-osmotic	Pseudohyponatremia (hyperlipidemia and hyperproteinemia), isotonic infusions, laboratory error	Correct lipids and protein levels
Hyperosmotic	Hyperglycemia or hypertonic infusions	Correct hyperglycemia[a] discontinue hypertonic fluids
Hypo-osmotic		
Hypovolemic–hypo-osmotic	Urine Na^+ >20: renal losses: RTA, adrenal insufficiency, diuretics, partial obstruction Urine Na^+ <10: extrarenal losses: vomiting, diarrhea, skin and lung loss, pancreatitis	Na^+ deficit[b] replaced as isotonic saline
Euvolemic–hypo-osmotic	H_2O intoxication, renal failure, syndrome of inappropriate antidiuretic hormone Hypothyroidism, pain drugs, adrenal insufficiency	Water restriction
Hypervolemic–hypo-osmotic	Urine Na^+ <10: nephritic syndrome, congestive heart failure, cirrhosis Urine Na^+ >20: iatrogenic volume overload, acute/chronic renal failure	Water restriction

[a] Corrected sodium = .016 (measured glucose − 100) + measured Na^+.
[b] Sodium deficit = (0.6 × weight in kg) × (140 − Na^+).

and management of specific types of hyponatremia are listed in Table 6.

Hypernatremia is defined as serum sodium greater than 145 mEq/L. The signs and symptoms of hypernatremia are listed in Box 4.

Spasticity

The neurologic symptoms of hypernatremia result from dehydration of brain cells. Laboratory tests used to diagnose hypernatremia are SUN and Cr, urine Na^+, and urine osmolality. A fluid deprivation test may be performed to distinguish central from nephrogenic diabetes insipidus. The etiology and management of specific types of hypernatremia are listed in Table 7. The rate of correction of plasma osmolality should not exceed 2 mOsm/kg/h. Overly aggressive correction may lead to central pontine myelinolysis.

Normal serum potassium level is 3.5 to 5.1 mEq/L. Hypokalemia is defined as serum potassium less than 3.5 mEq/L. Signs and symptoms associated with hypokalemia are listed in Box 5. Box 6 lists the major causes of hypokalemia.

Box 4. Signs and symptoms of hypernatremia

Confusion
Lethargy
Coma
Seizures
Hyperreflexia

Table 7
Etiology and management of hypernatremia

Hypernatremia	Etiology	Treatment
Hypervolemic	Administration of hypertonic sodium-containing solutions, mineralocorticoid excess	Diuretics
Isovolemic	Insensible skin and respiratory loss, diabetes insipidus	Water replacement[a]
Hypovolemic	Renal losses, gastrointestinal losses, respiratory losses, profuse sweating, adrenal deficiencies	Isotonic NaCl, then hypotonic saline

[a] Free water deficit = (.6 × weight in kg) × [(Na^+/140) − 1]. Half of the free water deficit is corrected over the first 24 hours. The rate of correction should not exceed .5–1 mEq/L/h.

> **Box 5. Signs and symptoms of hypokalemia**
>
> *Neuromuscular*
>
>   Muscle weakness
>   Paralysis
>   Rhabdomyolysis
>   Hyporeflexia
>
> *Gastrointestinal*
>
>   Paralytic ileus
>
> *Renal*
>
>   Polyuria
>   Polydipsia
>
> *Cardiac*
>
>   EKG findings: T-wave flattening/inversion
>   U-wave, ST depression
>   Cardiac toxicity to digitalis

> **Box 7. Signs and symptoms of hyperkalemia**
>
> *Neuromuscular*
>
>   Weakness
>   Paresthesia
>   Flaccid paralysis
>
> *Cardiac*
>
>   EKG findings: peaked T waves, flattened P waves, prolonged PR, widened QRS
>   Ventricular fibrillation
>   Cardiac arrest

A serum potassium level of 3 mEq/L indicates a potassium deficit of 250 mEq. A serum potassium level of 2 mEq/L represents a potassium deficit of over 700 mEq/L. Treatment for hypokalemia initially is aimed at correcting the existing metabolic abnormalities. Potassium chloride is administered at 10 mEq/L/h peripherally or 20 mEq/L/h centrally if EKG changes are present. Hypokalemia alone rarely produces cardiac arrhythmias.

Hyperkalemia is defined as serum potassium greater than 5.1 mEq/L. Signs and symptoms of hyperkalemia are listed in Box 7. Box 8 lists the common causes of hyperkalemia. Table 8 lists the options for the treatment of hyperkalemia.

Calcium

Normal calcium concentration is 8.8 to 10.5 mg/dL. The normal range for ionized calcium is 1.1 to 1.28 mg/dL. Calcium concentrations must be interpreted with respect to the serum albumin, because 40% to 60% of total serum calcium is bound to albumin: corrected calcium = ([4-albumin] × .8) + calcium $_{(serum)}$.

Because serum albumin does not affect the free unbound calcium (which is the active form), ionized calcium concentrations may be ordered, instead. Hypocalcemia is defined as serum calcium less than 8.5 mg/dL. Signs and symptoms of hypocalcemia are hypotension, larngeal spasm, paresthesias, tetany (Chvostek's and Trousseau's signs), anxiety, depression, and psychosis. In adults who have normal renal function, calcium replacement is 1 g (gluconate or chloride) in 50 mL dextrose 5% in water or normal saline. Intravenous solutions should be infused for 30 minutes.

> **Box 6. Causes of hypokalemia**
>
>   Decreased dietary intake
>   Gastrointestinal losses
>   Renal losses
>
>   Cellular shifts

> **Box 8. Causes of hyperkalemia**
>
>   Pseudohyperkalemia
>   Transcellular shift
>   Impaired renal excretion
>   Excessive intake
>   Blood transfusions

Table 8
Treatment of hyperkalemia

Treatment	Dosage	Rationale
Calcium gluconate	10–30 mL in 10% solution intravenously	Membrane stabilization
Sodium bicarbonate	50 mEq intravenously	Shifts K$^+$ into cells
Glucose-insulin	1 ampule D50 with 5 U regular insulin	Shifts K$^+$ into cells
Sodium polysterence Sulfonate	50–100 g enema with 50 mL 70% sorbitol and 100 mL water, or 20–40 g orally	Removes excess K$^+$ through gastrointestinal tract
Dialysis		Removes K$^+$ from serum

Hypercalcemia is serum calcium greater than 10.5 mg/dL. The signs and symptoms of hypercalcemia include hypertension, bradycardia, constipation, anorexia, nausea, vomiting, nephrolithiasis, bone pain, psychosis, and pruritus. Treatments include hydration with normal saline, bisphoshonates, calcitonin, glucocorticoids, and phosphate.

Magnesium

Magnesium concentration in the extracellular fluid ranges from 1.5 to 2.4 mg/dL. Uncorrected magnesium deficiencies impair repletion of cellular potassium and calcium. Hypomagnesemia is greater than 1.8 mg/dL. Signs and symptoms include arrhythmias, prolonged PR and QT intervals on EKG, hyperreflexia, fasciculations, and Chvostek's and Trousseau's signs. Guidelines for magnesium replacement are listed in Table 9.

Hypermagnesemia is serum mangensium greater than 2.3 mg/dL. Signs and symptoms include respiratory depression, hypotension, cardiac arrest, nausea and vomiting, hyporeflexia, and somnolence. Treatment for hypermagnesemia may include calcium infusion, saline infusion with a loop diuretic, or dialysis.

Table 9
Magnesium replacement

Magnesium serum concentration	Magnesium dosages
<1.5 mg/dl	1 mEq/kg
1.5–1.8 mg/dl	.5 mEq/kg

Table 10
Phosphorus replacement

Mild (2.3–3.0 mg/dL)	Moderate (1.6–2.2 mg/dL)	Severe (<1.5 mg/dL)
.16 mm/kg over 4–6 h	.32 mm/kg over 4–6 h	.64 mm over 8–12 h
Diluted in at least 100 mL	Dilute in at least 10 mL	Dilute in at least 100 mL

Phosphate

Normal phosphorus level is 2.5 to 4.9 mg/dL. Hypophosphatemia is serum phosphate less than 2.5 mg/dL; however, symptomatic hypophosphatemia usually is less than 1 mg/dL. Signs and symptoms of hypophosphatemia include lethargy, hypotension, irritability, cardiac arrhythmias, and skeletal demineralization. One millimeter of phosphate supplies 1.33 mEq sodium or 1.47 mEq potassium. Guidelines for phosphorus replacement in adults with adequate renal function are listed in Table 10.

Hyperphosphatemia is defined as serum phosphate greater than 5 mg/dL. Pruritus is the only remarkable symptom of hyperphosphatemia. Treatment includes dietary phosphate restriction, phosphate binders (calcium acetate or carbonate), hydration (to promote excretion), or D50 and insulin to shift phophate into cells.

Anticipation of blood product usage

A 75-kg male has approximately 48 liters of total body fluids, of which nearly 5 liters is whole blood. Table 11 details body fluid and blood volumes based on gender [3].

The allowable blood loss should be calculated preoperatively for patients in whom severe bleeding may be expected. Allowable blood loss (ABL) is

Table 11
Body fluid and blood volumes

Fluid	Men	Women
Total body fluid	600 mL/kg	500 mL/kg
Whole blood	66 mL/kg	60 mL/kg
Plasma	40 mL/kg	36 mL/kg
Erythrocytes	26 mL/kg	24 mL/kg

determined by the following formula: ABL = (estimated blood volume × [$H_i - H_f$]) ÷ H_i, where estimated blood volume = weight (kg) × average blood volume, H_i is the initial hematocrit, and H_f is the final acceptable hematocrit. The final acceptable hematocrit usually is 30% less than the initial hematocrit but varies according to individual circumstances. For example, for a 75-kg man who has an initial hematocrit of 45 g/dL, ABL = (4.95 L × [45 g/dL − 31.5 g/dL]) ÷ 45 g/dL = 1.485 L. This formula estimates allowable hemodilution, and accounts for ongoing replacement during surgery with either crystalloids or colloid fluids.

If patients are obese, using the ideal body weight (IBW) or adjusted body weight (ABW) to determine estimated blood volume gives more accuracy than actual body weight. The IBW in kilograms is determined as follows: men—IBW = 50 kg + 2.3 kg for each inch over 5 feet; women—IBW = 45.5 kg + 2.3 kg for each inch over 5 feet.

If actual body weight is 30% greater than the calculated IBW, calculate the ABW. The ABW is calculated as follows: ABW = IBW + .4 × (actual weight − IBW).

Therefore, for obese patients, the allowable blood loss is calculated using the following formula: ABL = ([ABW × ABV] × [$H_i - H_f$]) ÷ H_i.

For example, to calculate the ABL for a 5′2″ woman who weighs 110 kg and has an initial hematocrit of 40 g/dL:

IBW = 50 kg + 4.6 kg = 54.6 kg
 (110 kg is 49.6% > 54.6, so use ABW)

ABW = 54.6 × .4(110 − 54.6) = 32 kg

ABL = ([32 kg × 60 mL/kg] × [40 g/dL − 28 g/dL])
 ÷ 40 g/dL = .576 L

The route of vascular access must be considered preoperatively. The dimensions of the vascular catheter determine the rate of volume infusion. According to the Hagen-Poiseuille equation (which describes flow through rigid tubes), if the radius of a catheter is doubled, the flow rate through the catheter increases 16-fold [4]. Furthermore, as the length of the catheter is doubled, the infusion rate decreases by one half. Therefore, because central venous catheters are 2 to 3 times longer than peripheral angiocatheters, given equal gauges, a peripheral venous catheter is preferable for volume resuscitation.

Prevention of fluid imbalances may be achieved by the application of basic maneuvers and the adherence to fundamental principles. For surgeries in the head and neck region, the reverse Trendelenburg position is a simple maneuver to decrease blood loss. Hypotensive anesthesia (commonly used for maxillary osteotomies) is another useful adjunct. A 20% reduction in preoperative blood pressure is shown to result in a 40% reduction in operative blood loss. In addition, the use of agents locally (epinephrine) or topically (thrombin-soaked sponges, gelfoam, or oxidized cellulose) can prevent or control significant hemorrhage.

Volume resuscitation

When blood loss is mild (less than 15% of blood volume), no volume resuscitation is necessary. With moderate to severe blood loss, the vascular space must be filled to support cardiac output. Although it often is used for hypovolemic hypotension, the Trendelenburg position does not promote venous return, and, hence, does not increase cardiac output [5]. The only effective management of hypovolemia is volume resuscitation. Crystalloid fluids may be used for volume resuscitation. Because crystalloids cross plasma membranes readily, the volume of crystalloid fluid administration must be 3 times the volume of the estimated blood loss. Alternatively, colloids may be used for volume resuscitation. Colloids are large molecules that do not diffuse across membranes readily. Colloids are efficient plasma expanders. Box 9 lists the commonly used colloids.

Rapid intravascular volume expansion is accomplished best with 5% albumin. The primary indication for 25% albumin is hypoalbuminmia. Plasma protein fractions (PPF) are used for the treatment of hypoproteinemia. The disadvantage of PPF administration is that it may result in hypotension secondary to decreased systemic vascular resistance. The administration of hetastarch and dextran in large volumes can result in dilutional coagulopathies. Hetastarch, when administered in greater than 1000 mL (in a 70-kg patient), can precipitate a decrease in factor VIII. Dextran can decrease platelet

> **Box 9. Plasma expanders**
>
> *Human albumin*
>
>   Albutein 5%
>   Albutein 25%
>   Albuminar-5
>   Albuminar-25
>   Buminate 5%
>   Buminate 25%
>
> *Plasma protein fractions: albumin 4.4%*
>
>   Plasmanate
>   Plamatein
>   Plasma-Plex
>   Proteinate
>
> *Dextrans and starch*
>
>   Dextran 40
>   Dextran 70
>   Hetastarch

> **Box 10. Method for determining resuscitation volume sequence**
>
> 1. Estimate normal blood volume
> 2. Estimate percent loss of blood volume
> 3. Calculate volume deficit
> 4. Determine resuscitation volume

adhesiveness and may cause an anaphylactoid or anaphylactic reaction. In addition, dextran also facilitates the agglutination of red blood cells. Therefore, dextran administration interferes with the subsequent crossmatching of blood. Colloids are administered at a 1:1 ratio to replace blood loss.

Indications for blood therapy

The indication for blood transfusion is to increase the oxygen-carrying capacity of the blood. Blood transfusion almost always is indicated for hemoglobin less than 6 g/dL. Because oxygen transport is maximal at hemoglobin levels above 10 g/dL, blood transfusion rarely is justified for hemoglobin values greater than 10 g/dL. The decision to transfuse blood, however, never is based solely on the hemoglobin concentration, but rather within the context of the complete clinical presentation, accounting for modifying factors, such as age and medical status, the surgical procedure, and anticipation of ongoing losses exceeding 100 mL/min. Clinical signs of blood loss include hypotension, tachycardia, and oliguria.

The American College of Surgeons describes four categories of acute blood loss (Table 12) [6].

Acute loss of volumes greater than 40% of patients' total blood volume or acute loss leading to hypovolemic shock usually necessitates blood transfusion. In hypovolemic shock, a standard volume resuscitation approach is to administer 2 liters of crystalloid fluid as a bolus. If a favorable response is not obtained, then colloid fluids are added to the regimen. Box 10 shows a logical method for volume resuscitation.

Volume deficit is calculated by multiplying the estimated blood volume by the percent of blood loss. There is a 1:1 ratio of colloid replacement to blood loss and a 3:1 ratio for crystalloid replacement.

Table 12
Classification of acute hemorrhage

Parameter	Class I	Class II	Class III	Class IV
% loss of blood volume	<15%	15%–30%	30%–40%	>40%
Pulse rate	<100	>100	>120	>140
Blood pressure	Normal	Normal	Decreased	Normal
Urine output (mL/h)	>30	20–30	5–15	<5

Blood component therapy

Transfusion with whole blood rarely is indicated. Components obtained from whole blood include packed red blood cells, platelet concentrates, fresh frozen plasma, cryoprecipitate, factor VIII, albumin, PPF, leukocyte-poor blood, and antibody concentrates. Blood components are preferable to whole blood for several reasons. Component therapy allows specific deficiencies to be addressed, preserves the remaining whole blood components, allows longer storage, and reduces the risk for transfusion reaction. The American Red Cross has indication guidelines

Table 13
Indication guidelines for the most commonly administered blood components

Component	Indications
Red blood cells	Symptomatic chronic anemia in normovolemic patients, if pharmacologic therapy is not effective or available
	Prophylactic transfusion to prevent morbidity from anemia patients at greater risk for tissue hypoxia
	Active bleeding, with signs and symptoms of hypovolemia unresponsive to crystalloid or colloid infusions
	Preoperative anemia <9 g/dL with impending major blood loss
	Sickle cell disease
	Anemia due to renal failure or hemodialysis refractory to erythropoietin therapy
Platelets	Prevention or treatment of nonsurgical bleeding due to thrombocytopenia
	Patients who have accelerated platelet destruction with significant bleeding
	Prior to surgical and major invasive procedures when the platelet count is <50,000 μL
	Diffuse microvascular bleeding after massive transfusion
Fresh frozen plasma	Bleeding, preoperative, or massively transfused patients with a deficiency of multiple coagulation factors
	Patients who have bleeding or urgent invasive procedures on warfarin therapy
	Thrombotic thrombocytopenic purpura and related syndromes
	Congenital or acquired coagulation factor deficiency when no concentrate is available
	Specific plasma protein deficiencies
Cryoprecipitate	Treatment of bleeding due to hypofibrinogenemia or dysfibriginomeia
	Cases of disseminated intravascular coagulation when fibrinogen and factor VIII may be depleted
	Prophylaxis or treatment of significant factor XIII deficiency
Factor VIII	Treatment of hemophilia A
	Treatment of von Willebrand's disease

for the most commonly administered blood components (Table 13) [7].

Complications of blood product usage

The complications associated with blood product usage include transfusion reactions, metabolic abnormalities, microaggregates, hypothermia, coagulation disorders, and acute lung injury. Treatments for the various blood product usage complications are listed in Table 14.

Autologous blood usage

Autologous blood donation is possible for healthy patients scheduled for surgery in whom significant blood loss is expected. A common collection protocol is donation of 1 unit of blood every 4 days for a maximum of 3 units. The last unit must be donated no sooner than 72 hours before the surgery to restore plasma volume.

Intraoperative blood salvage involves the collection, washing, and storage of red blood cells by a semiautomated system. The hematocrit of salvaged blood is between 50% and 60%, and the pH is alkaline. Contraindications to intraoperative blood salvage include blood-borne diseases, malignancy, and contamination.

Hemodilution involves the removal of arterial or venous blood preoperatively, followed by plasma volume restoration with crystalloid or colloid fluids. The blood then is stored in the operating room and transfused to the patient after cessation of bleeding. This procedure may be used for surgeries in which intraoperative blood loss of 2 or more units is anticipated.

End parameters of volume resuscitation

The primary goal of volume resuscitation is the restoration of oxygen uptake into the vital organs to sustain aerobic metabolism. The major determinants of oxygen uptake are cardiac output and hemoglobin. Blood products do not increase blood flow adequately and in some cases impede flow as a result of increased viscosity. Therefore, crystalloid and colloid fluids should be the initial management

Table 14
Complications associated with blood product usage

Complication	Sign/symptoms	Treatment/prevention
Transfusion reaction		
Febrile	Fever, chills, headache myalgias, nausea, nonproductive cough	Antipyretics
Allergic	Urticaria, pruritus, facial swelling	Intravenous antihistamines
Hemolytic	Fever, chills, chest pain, chest pain, nausea, flushing dyspnea, hypotension, hemoglobinuria	Stop transfusion; Lactated Ringer's/ mannitol/furosemide
Coagulation disorder		
Dilutional Thrombocytopenia	Lack of blood-clotting ability	Platelets
Factor V and VIII deficiency	Prolonged PT/PTT	FFP
Disseminated intravascular coagulation	Prolonged PT/PTT, increased fibrin split products, decreased serum fibrinogen	Platelets/FFP
Metabolic abnormality		
Hyperkalemia	Weakness, paresthesias, flaccid paralysis, elevated T wave	Calcium gluconate, calcium chloride, insulin-dextrose, loop diuretics, hemodialysis
Hypocalcemia	Hypotension, narrow pulse pressure, hyperreflexia, prolonged QT interval, tetany, shortened PR interval	Calcium gluconate, Calcium chloride
Metabolic alkalosis	Muscle cramps, weakness, hypoxia, arrhythmias	None required; Usually self-correcting
Hypothermia	Cardiac irritability, shivering, increased myocardial oxygen demand	Warm blood to 38°; Prior to Tx
Acute lung injury	Noncardiogenic pulmonary edema, dyspnea, hypoxemia	Supportive
Microaggregates	Vascular obstruction, fever	Micropore filters

strategy for volume resuscitation in acute hemorrhage. Blood gas analysis and central venous pressure or pulmonary artery monitoring yield useful information regarding volume status. The goals of volume resuscitation based on hemodynamic monitoring and blood gas analysis are listed in Box 11 [8].

Ultimately, the clinical indicators that are readily observable determine the end parameters of volume resuscitation. A favorable clinical response includes adequate blood pressure and heart rate, urine output greater than 1 mL/kg/h, and adequate oxygen saturation.

Surgical management and medical management of oral and maxillofacial surgery patients are intertwined intimately. The management of fluids and electrolytes and the usage of blood products are governed by the basic principles outlined in this article. It is incumbent on oral and maxillofacial surgeons to have a thorough understanding of the surgical and medical issues that face patients. A favorable surgical outcome is predicated on optimal comprehensive care.

Box 11. Goals of volume resuscitation

1. Central venous pressure = 15 mm Hg
2. Pulmonary capillary wedge pressure = 10 to 12 mm Hg
3. Cardiac index > 3 L/min/m^2
4. Oxygen uptake (Vo$_2$) > 100 mL/min/m^2
5. Blood lactate < 4 mmol/L
6. Base deficit − 3 to + 3 mmol/L

References

[1] Shires III GT, Barber A, Shires GT. Fluid and electrolyte management of the surgical patient. In: Shires GT, editor. Schwartz's principles of surgery. 7th ed. Philadelphia: McGraw-Hill; 1999. p. 53–74.

[2] Wait RB, Kim KU, Isha MA. Fluid, electrolytes, and acid-base balance. In: Greenfield LJ, et al, editors. Surgery scientific principles of practice. 3rd ed. Philadelphia: Lippincott Williams and Wilkins; 2001. p. 244–69.

[3] Skeie B, Askanzai J, Khambatta H. Nutrition, fluid, and electrolytes. In: Barash PG, editor. Clincial anesthesia. 4th ed. Lippincott Williams and Wilkins; 2001. p. 721–51.
[4] Dula DJ, Lutz P, Vogel MF, et al. Rapid flow rates for the resuscitation of hypovolemic shock. Ann Emerg Med 1985;14:303–6.
[5] Sing R, O'Hara D, Sawyer MA, et al. Trendelenburg position and oxygen transport in hypovolemic adults. Ann Emerg Med 1994;23:564–8.
[6] Committee on Trauma. Advanced trauma life support student manual. 6th ed. Chicago: American College of Surgeons; 2001. p. 87–107.
[7] The American Red Cross. Blood components medical update. Dedham (MA): American Red Cross Blood Services, New England Region; 2001.
[8] Marino PL. Hemorrhage and hypovolemia. In: The ICU book. 2nd ed. Baltimore: Williams and Wilkins; 1998. p. 207–27.

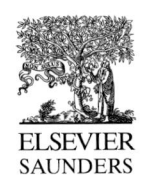

Perioperative Risk Assessment in the Surgical Care of Geriatric Patients

Leslie R. Halpern, DDS, MD, PhD, MPH[a,b,*], Seth Feldman, DDS[b,c]

[a]*Department of Oral and Maxillofacial Surgery, Massachusetts General Hospital, Boston, MA, USA*
[b]*Harvard School of Dental Medicine, Boston, MA, USA*
[c]*Cambridge Health Alliance, Cambridge, MA, USA*

The geriatric population comprises an increasing percentage of the overall population in the United States. Currently 13.6% of the population is age 65 or older, and 6% are 80 or older [1]. The importance of oral health within the geriatric sector has been given more recognition, because there is a synergistic relationship between oral health and overall health. Advances in surgical and anesthetic techniques combined with sophisticated perioperative monitoring are factors that have contributed to an expanding number of older adults undergoing oral surgery. The elderly often have multiple comorbid conditions limiting their functional capacity to withstand the stress of surgery and postoperative recovery. As such, surgical management becomes more challenging and the role of oral and maxillofacial surgeons becomes paramount. It involves clinical competency and ability to evaluate carefully the pathophysiologic risk of comorbid disease in order to provide safe, expedient, and effective surgical care.

This review paper attempts to focus on the importance of perioperative risk assessment when applying oral surgical therapeutics to geriatric patients. Specifically, medical workup of comorbid systemic illnesses and pharmacologic therapy are assessed in order to determine appropriate treatment strategies for successful surgical outcomes.

General medical history and informed consent

Retrospective studies, using hospital database chart reviews, have examined the predictor variables of age and severity of illness in geriatric surgical patients on outcome and length of hospital stay. When age and severity of illness are compared, the severity of illness provides a better predictor of surgical outcome and length of hospital stay [2–4]. As such, the perioperative assessment of elderly patients should begin the moment they enter the office. A first impression of a patient's physical appearance, gait, posture, attitude, and behavior should be noted [5]. Many practitioners find inconsistencies when history forms are filled out in the waiting area and then are reviewed prior to treatment planning [6]. Medical consultations must be undertaken judiciously for patients whose medical histories are uncertain and when the physical assessment uncovers an untreated medical problem.

A thorough preoperative workup includes medical, social, and cognitive history; physical examination; laboratory profile; and nutritional status.

Nutrition and fluid electrolytes

Nutritional deficits of a multifactorial etiology are most prevalent in elderly surgical patients. Risk factors for malnutrition either are macronutrient (protein, fats, and carbohydrates) or micronutrient (vitamins and minerals) in origin. In addition, malnutrition can be iatrogenic as a result of adverse drug-nutrient interactions, causing a depletion of daily

---

* Corresponding author. Department of Oral and Maxillofacial Surgery, Massachusetts General Hospital, Warren 1201, 55 Fruit Street, Boston, MA 02114.
 E-mail address: lhalpern1@partners.org (L.R. Halpern).

needed elements as a trade-off for treatment of systemic illnesses [7]. Perioperative risk assessment of nutritional status requires clinical, biochemical, anthropometric, and dietary monitoring strategies. Specifically, rapid weight loss greater than 10% should be of concern. Laboratory panels should be ordered to characterize the severity of malnutrition [7–9]. Protein energy malnutrition is most common and arises from a deficit in serum albumin [10]. Postoperative sequelae in patients who have protein energy malnutrition include poor wound healing, increased wound infection, and risk of mortality. Albumin levels of less than 3.2 g/dL in hospitalized older persons are highly predictive of subsequent mortality [8]. Cholesterol levels of less than 160 mg/dL in frail elderly persons also are a risk marker for increased mortality [9]. Complete blood cell counts should include a total lymphocyte count (no less than 1500/μL) and anergy skin testing. Although the latter have not proved useful nutritional markers in older persons, these predictors must be considered, because the elderly population often suffers from opportunistic infections and delayed healing resulting from chronic diseases, such as diabetes and peripheral vascular disease [8,10].

Specific nutritional supplements for proteins and kilocalorie replacement should be prescribed preoperatively and during the perioperative period. Common protein supplement recommendations are Ensure/Ensure Plus (Abbott Labs, Abbott Park, IL) and Sustacal (Mead Johnson, Evansville, IN) along with resuming a well-balanced diet as tolerated. Postoperative laboratory analyses, using the criteria described previously, allow for immediate resolution of any physiologic imbalances that can impede surgical recovery [9]. Postsurgical care should include nutritional counseling with dietary suggestions that can be understood easily and reinforced at follow-up visits. Postoperative planning includes a team approach with a general dental practitioner, because loss of teeth or poor-fitting dentures contribute significantly to malnutrition and depression, with resultant weight loss in these patients.

Fluid and electrolyte balance play a pivotal role in perioperative surgical risk assessment. With aging, there are increases in total body fat and decreases in total body water. Both can contribute to an imbalance in fluids and electrolytes. Decreased urinary concentrating ability; limitations in excretion of water, sodium, and potassium; and "iatrogenic injury" with intravenous fluid overload can exacerbate trauma to tissues further and alter the hemodynamic state of patients [11]. Furthermore, impaired thirst perception, decreased glomerular filtration rate, and alterations in hormonal levels of antidiuretic hormone, atrial natriuretic peptide, and aldosterone can initiate or exacerbate the systemic neurologic and cardiovascular complications of hyperkalemia, hypernatremia, and volume depletion and the complication of postoperative delirium (discussed later) [11].

Strategies to preventive imbalances include perioperative measurements of serum electrolytes, urea nitrogen, serum creatinine, and creatinine clearance and a baseline urinalysis. Normal fluid management should be maintained in a range of 1.5 to 2.0 L/d with an average urine output of 20 to 30 mL/h [11]. Elderly patients who have undergone uncomplicated dentoalveolar surgery are encouraged to resume oral intake as soon as possible in order to maintain fluid and electrolyte balance. Patients who may vomit or develop severe diarrhea after surgery also should be monitored, because metabolic acidosis or alkalosis can precipitate the adverse events of delirium and cardiac dysrhythmias. Patients who are in the postoperative phase after general anesthesia must be monitored for ongoing fluid losses from all sites, including insensible losses. Adverse drug effects from postoperative "polypharmaceutical administration" also can alter salt and water balance. The adequacy of free-water replacement should be guided by the serum electrolyte concentration gradients with judicious monitoring to prevent these events. Dehydration is seen more often than overhydration and it may be wise to maintain fluids and electrolytes parentally along with monitoring vital signs preoperatively and postoperatively.

Social history

Social history and lifestyle issues, especially use of tobacco and alcohol, need to be documented. Cessation of smoking can be accomplished even in geriatric patients. Studies suggest that elderly patients should refrain from tobacco use up to 6 months prior to any surgical procedures [12]. Alcohol consumption is associated with complex changes in cerebral vasculature and structure in older adults. Often, alcohol abuse is misdiagnosed and the cause of falls and accidents. It also is associated with severe malnutrition, poor wound healing, and decreased immune competence. The role of alcohol consumption and the incidence of dementia are less clear but often considered in the elderly. Studies suggest that participants who drink no alcohol at midlife and those who drank alcohol frequently are twice as likely to have mild cognitive impairment in old age as those participants who drink alcohol infrequently [13]. Preoperative risk assessment with the CAGE protocol or use of laboratory tests (discussed previously) allow surgeons to determine if patients need any prophylaxis for complications of alcoholism withdrawal during the perioperative period.

Cognitive evaluation and informed consent

Cognitive assessment and the ability to give informed consent are of major concern when evaluating geriatric patients for surgery. Simple questions can evaluate patients' orientation to time and place and ability to recall information, perform simple calculations, or understand speech. Doctors should speak directly to patients when reviewing health history and should make sure the wording is understood, because many patients have hearing and visual impairments [6,14]. Many patients do not admit readily that they did not understand questions. Although modifying the history-taking by including family members and caregivers may be considered, it is important to remember that even cognitively impaired patients can provide useful information if the questions are presented in a concrete and simple manner. Decision capacity should be predicated on formal mental status criteria in order to judge whether or not patients are capable of receiving informed consent. Patients can be lucid during specific periods of time but not others (sundowning) and still be able to give informed consent. If patients cannot provide informed consent, alternative choices include written documents for power of attorney by chosen executors or power of living wills [15].

Medications

The physiologic and pathologic changes occurring in older patients can lead to adverse events with respect to medications taken. Blood flow to the liver decreases with age and the bioavailability of drugs can be altered depending on their metabolic pathway [16]. Renal clearance is altered significantly with age because of the morphologic decrease in mass associated with decreased tubular function and glomerular filtration rate. Other systemic factors can affect the distribution of drugs in the elderly, such as decreased cardiac output, increased peripheral vascular resistance, and increases in percentage of adipose tissue in the body [17,18]. Other organ functions can be affected, such as the digestive system, gastric acid production, and gastric emptying time. It is not unusual for patients to be taking from 4 to 8 other medications depending on their degree of chronic illnesses. Surgeons must be judicious in cataloguing all drugs prior to beginning treatment. Patients often may not remember the names of all the medications they are taking, and a medical consultation is necessary to obtain an accurate list. The most common types of medications that the elderly take are over-the-counter (OTC) medications for pain and other chronic ailments.

Over-the-counter drugs

Data shows that only 11% of physicians ask routinely about OTC drug use during primary care visits [13]. It is important to discuss the use of nonprescription medications with elderly patients, because adverse effects can be seen when combined with any prescribed agents during the perioperative period. Many geriatric patients forget to write the type and number of OTC drugs on the history form. The most common ailment for which 66% of the elderly use OTC drugs is arthritis and the most common medications used are acetaminophen, aspirin, or other nonsteroidal anti-inflammatory drugs (NSAIDs). Other OTC drugs used on a daily basis include a variety of gastrointestinal agents, such as antacids and H_2-blockers, both of which can interfere with medications adversely for cardiovascular function (ie, anticoagulants and antiarrhythmia agents, such as digoxin, lidocaine, and procainamide). Surgeons must educate patients and their caregivers carefully on side effects and emphasize cautiousness when they use OTC drugs. In addition, medicines should be catalogued and dated so that patients do not take any expired drugs that can exacerbate side effects.

Pain control

Strategies for pain management must be orchestrated carefully, because the central nervous system–depressant effects of analgesic medication can initiate or exacerbate the postoperative depression and delirium observed when the elderly undergo surgical treatment. The main first-line choices for mild to moderate pain are aspirin and acetaminophen. The preferred choice for pain relief is acetaminophen (200 to 400 mg every 4 to 6 hours with a maximum of 1.2 grams per day) [17]. Acetaminophen with codeine is useful when used with appropriate precaution. Pain that is more severe requires the administration of narcotics. Each narcotic should be prescribed based on the individual. Side effects of confusion, respiratory depression, and constipation should be weighed against the benefits of the drug [17,18].

Aspirin should be used with caution, because it can potentiate bleeding resulting from altered platelet function and increased capillary fragility in the elderly. NSAIDs may be an alternative when patients are unable to tolerate a narcotic. Advantages include the avoidance of respiratory depression, peripheral activity, and minimal neural side effects. Disadvantages include increased fluid retention, renal failure, hepatotoxicity, gastrointestinal ulceration, and respiratory compromise in patients sensitive to aspirin or aspirin-like products [19,20].

Other centrally acting agents are suggested, such as tramadol (Ultram). It can be used to treat moderate to severe pain and is the drug of choice for patients who have malignant pain [21].

Dosing for moderate to severe pain can vary from 50 to 100 mg every 4 to 6 hours with a maximum dose of 400 mg per day. Side effects include nausea, dizziness, seizures, and somnolence. Careful choices, therefore, must be made with respect to the patients who would benefit from this pain medication [22].

Sedation strategies for elderly surgical patients

The ideal sedative should have some basic requirements that permit safety to the recipient and provide operating conditions that permit high-quality surgical intervention [23,24]. Sedation techniques usually are based on the nature and severity of specific risk factors, such as comorbid systemic illnesses [25,26]. Basic criteria for the use of sedation in the elderly are listed in Box 1. The methods of sedation used most often in geriatric patients to treat pain and anxiety are oral, inhalation, and intravenous approaches and general anesthesia. Each method applies the adjunctive use of local anesthesia for pain control [27].

Box 1. Criteria for sedation in the elderly

- Refusal of care
- Unpredictable behavior patterns
- Health problems exacerbated by stress
- Noncompliance and inability to obey instructions
- Danger of hurting themselves
- Aggressiveness while under therapy

Adapted from Matear DW, Clarke D. Considerations for the use of oral sedation in the institutionalized geriatric patient during dental interventions: a review of the literature. Special Care Dent 1999;19:56–63.

Local anesthesia

Local anesthetic administration at low doses often is the preferred method for pain management in the elderly. Careful titration always is prudent, because there can be cardiovascular responses to epinephrine-containing anesthetic agents [27]. There are few incidences of hypersensitivity or allergic reactions to local anesthetics and few adverse effects with normal dosage on the cardiovascular or respiratory system. For these patients, generally, not more than 2×1.8 mL carpules of 2% Lidocaine with 1:100,000 epinephrine should be used for anesthesia, because minimal cardiac side effects are seen with this dosage [17]. The body produces endogenous epinephrine in far greater amounts in response to a stressful situation, which can occur during surgical procedures. During deeper sedation, the recommended doses of epinephrine are limited further in the elderly in order to avoid arrhythmias and hypertensive episodes [17,27].

Inhalation sedation with nitrous oxide

Nitrous oxide is a safe method for pain and anxiety management in the elderly because of its rapid elimination and nondepressant effect on cardiovascular function. It is noninvasive, titratable, and easily reversible. Patient acceptance, cost, ease of use, rapid onset, and rapid elimination make it preferable to oral and intravenous sedation. Retrospective cross-sectional studies show that a majority of patients, young and older, have fair acceptance to the use of nitrous oxide for pain and anxiety [28]. Careful preoperative assessment should include a cognitive examination, because the elderly are susceptible to bouts of dementia and may not be aware of their surroundings in order to cooperate [29].

Oral sedation

The use of oral sedation in the elderly is acceptable and often chosen for the reduction of preoperative pain and stress prior to and during surgical treatment. The advantages of using oral sedating agents include low cost, ease of administration, and decreased adverse reactions (depending on the oral agent). Disadvantages of oral sedation include patient compliance, frequent in the elderly, and the inability to properly dose or titrate the drug. The pharmacologic agents used most commonly include sedative hypnotics (such as barbiturates), antihistamines, narcotic analgesics, and benzodiazepines [23,30–32]. The first three drug groups often are contraindicated because of many side effects. Their use, however, can

> **Box 2. Criteria for the ideal benzodiazepine**
>
> - Rapid onset (ie, 15–30 minutes)
> - Short acting (ie, 30–60 minutes)
> - Rate of elimination less than 8–10 hours
> - Small titrating doses
> - No active metabolites
>
> *Adapted from* Leffler PM. Oral benzodiazepines and conscious sedation. J Oral Maxillofac Surg 1992;50:989–97.

be predicated upon careful titration in order to avoid hypotension, apnea, and unconsciousness resulting from cardiovascular compromise and respiratory depression (discussed later).

The benzodiazepines are the drug group of choice, because they have proved over time to be efficacious and safe when given to patients who are medically compromised and cognitively [26,30–32].

Box 2 describes the ideal benzodiazepine. Benzodiazepines may be given orally for anxiety control or intravenously as part of conscious sedation. These medications again are usually given in lower doses for the elderly because of decreased metabolism and clearance of the agents [30–32]. Diazepam (Valium), for example, has a long half-life and active metabolic products, which, in the presence of impaired metabolism and excretion of the drug, increase the likelihood and duration of possible side effects, such as confusion and gait instability. A benzodiazepine, such as triazolam (Halcion) or lorazepam (Ativan), with a shorter half-life, is a more appropriate choice [30]. Contraindications for triazolam use occur in patients who have a history of depression and glaucoma. In addition, patients who are on Phenytoin for seizures and depression and those who are on erythromycin antibiotics or who are suffering from degenerative neurologic disorders, such as myasthenia gravis, should not be given triazolam [30,32].

Table 1 compares the choices for oral sedation with dose and peak onset of action. Regardless of the choice of sedation drug, basic guidelines include a comprehensive preoperative medical history, familiarity with the sedation medication used, titration based on specific body morphometry and lowest dose needed, and, most important, ensuring that staff is trained properly in the event of an emergency. Patients who have any baseline disorientation must be assessed and observed overnight, because temporary postoperative delirium can occur in a large percentage of geriatric patients. Nothing-by-mouth status, immobilization, and the presence of midazolam also can increase the risk of postoperative delirium. Sensory aids, reorientation, and family contact are key in the prevention of delirium (postoperative delirium is discussed later) [31].

Intravenous sedation

Studies show that IV conscious sedation provides a clinical scenario in which healthy or disabled elderly patients can be treated safely and effectively [33–35]. Advantages of IV sedation include predictability, titratablity, rapid onset, patient acceptance, and reversibility. Disadvantages include difficulty in developing the technique, operator training, state and office requirements, monitoring and record keeping, cost with respect to operator and patient, and proper assistant training. The logistics of patient preparation entails a stepwise algorithm starting with the placement of the monitoring devises without undue stress. Continuous monitoring is required before, during, and after procedures. Recommended monitoring includes pulse oximetry, ECG, blood pressure monitoring, and a continuous recording of vital signs.

Table 1
A comparison of triazolam, oxazepam, and lorazepam for oral sedation

Sedating agent	Oral dosage[a]	Onset of action	Peak blood level
Triazolam (Halcion)	0.0625–0.125 mg	Within 30 minutes	30–120 minutes
Oxazepam (Serax)	10–30 mg	Within 60–120 minutes	120–240 minutes
Lorazepam (Ativan)	0.5–2.0 mg	Within 30–60 minutes	30–180 minutes

[a] Dosage: healthy adult doses are greater than 10 times the dose stated for elderly patients.
Adapted from Matear DW, Clarke D. Considerations for the use of oral sedation in the institutionalized geriatric patient during dental interventions: a review of the literature. Spec Care Dent 1999;19:56–63.

Extra padding should be placed on the dental chair to prevent compression sores. Placement of the catheter must be done with care, because the skin often is fragile and the veins can tear more easily with formation of a painful hematoma. Adhesive tape to stabilize the site must be positioned carefully so as to not tear the skin.

The half-life of many IV sedation drugs, such as fentanyl, diazepam, and midazolam, is increased significantly in older adults [33,34,36]. In the elderly, slower stepping of the dosage is recommended, allowing more time for peak effect under lower doses [35,36]. Table 2 lists acceptable dosing of sedation medications for IV procedures. These doses allow patients to maintain their own airway with little chance for significant respiratory complications [34,36]. Comprehensive postoperative monitoring must be administered during recovery time, because adverse effects of IV sedation include postoperative delirium and increased risk for falls and subsequent hospitalization [37].

General anesthesia

General anesthesia can be an alternative choice for elderly patients who are in excellent health or are no longer able to tolerate treatment safely in an outpatient setting. There are significant risks, however, to general anesthesia, including episodes of severe hypotension or hypertension, hypothermia, hypoxia, nausea, prolonged sedation or delirium, and even pneumonia, cardiac arrest, and death. A survey done in France from 1978 to 1982 indicates a tenfold increase in the rate of postoperative anesthetic complications as patients' ages increases from 30 to 80 years. The complication rate, however, when scrutinized, shows that the frequency of complications was 0.5% in ages greater than 80 [38]. A case series at the Mayo Clinic indicates a 9.4% morbidity rate in 795 patients 90 years of age and older and only one major complication in 31 patients' ages 100 to 107 [39]. Recent studies show a decline in the morbidity and mortality rates and the overall frequency of perioperative complications in the elderly who have undergone surgical procedures with general anesthesia [26,35]. Such data suggest that anesthetic management in the operating room should not be denied on the basis of age alone.

The preanesthetic evaluation of elderly patients is accomplished best a few days before the procedure. This allows a therapeutic alliance to develop between patient, anesthesiologist, and nursing and allied staff. Safety of anesthetic techniques can be discussed completely, which may reduce patient anxiety and preconceived negative beliefs of the morbidity associated with general anesthesia.

The choice of anesthetic agent is predicated on the specific cardiovascular status of patients [40]. In general, with age, there is a concomitant decrease in cardiac, vascular, and autonomic function. There also is a reduction in heart rate as a result of decreased β-adrenergic stimulation. This compromises the baroreflex-mediated increase in heart rate resulting from hypotension. The elderly subsequently have a greater decrease in blood pressure at a given concentration of volatile agent than younger patients [40,41]. Furthermore, the elderly are more susceptible to enhanced decreased myocardial contractility with volatile agents and any cardiac pathology already present is exacerbated. Most importantly, hemodynamic control may play a more important role in avoiding cardiovascular complications from general anesthetics, because many elderly exhibit a contracted volume state [41]. The choices of volatile agents most likely to maintain hemodynamic balance in the elderly are isoflurane and Desflurane [42]. Both are eliminated safely by pulmonary ventilation that avoids a compromise of hepatic and renal distribution. Desflurane seems to have a more rapid elimination and recovery time that improves cognitive function and decreased postanesthetic management [41,42].

The American Society of Anesthesiologists (ASA) suggests criteria for elderly patients who are being considered for general anesthesia [40]. These include and are not limited to:

1. Individuals older than 65 have, on average, 3.5 medical diseases that may be atypical on presentation.

Table 2
Recommended dosing for sedation with intravenous agents

	Midazolam	Diazepam	Meperidine
Malamed et al	1 0.1.5 mg/kg[a]	1.0 mg/kg[b]	N/A
Galli and Henry	2.0–2.5 mg/ 10–15[a] minute intervals	2 mg/10–15[c] minute intervals	1.0 mg/kg[b]

[a] Maximum dose of midazolam not to exceed 10 mg.
[b] Maximum dose of meperidine not to exceed 50 mg.
[c] Maximum dose of diazepam not to exceed 10 mg.

Adapted from Malamed SF, Gottschalk HW, Mulligan R, Quinn CL. Intravenous sedation for conservative dentistry for disabled patients. Anesth Prog 1989;36:140–2; and Galli MT, Henry RG. Using intravenous sedation to manage adults with neurological impairment. Spec Care Dent 1999; 19:275–80.

2. Significant interindividual variability exists among elderly patients when evaluating their medical diseases.
3. Unpredictability of diminished organ reserves is most apparent during surgery.
4. The impact of extrinsic factors (ie, smoking, alcohol, socioeconomic status, and environment) is difficult to quantify as predictors for successful outcome.
5. ASA status: ASA 1, age less than 70 years and nonemergent surgery; ASA II, patients more than 70 years; ASA III, patients who have comorbid illnesses and are treated in the hospital setting.

Risk assessment of comorbid systemic disease

Table 3 lists the common chronic illnesses seen within the geriatric population. The sections that follow discuss each comorbid disease with respect to its pathophysiology and offer suggestions for evaluation and treatment during the perioperative period.

Cardiovascular disease

A high prevalence of coronary artery disease and hypertension exists in the population at large, and heart disease accounts for 33% of deaths in adults over age 65 [43]. Common cardiovascular predictors of an adverse outcome include ischemic heart disease, dysrhythmias, congestive heart failure (CHF), peripheral vascular disease, and hypertension. The evaluation of patients' cardiac status begins with specific indications (ie, inability to walk less than 2 blocks; history of chest pain or jaw pain radiating to the left arm; unstable angina; history of CHF or pump failure

Table 3
Prevalence of chronic conditions in persons 70 years of age and older in the United States, 1995

Arthritis	56%
Hypertension	34%
Heart disease	25%
Diabetes	11%
Respiratory diseases	11%
Stroke	9%
Cancer	4%

Data from Centers for Disease Control and Prevention, National Center for Health Interview Survey, Second Supplement on Aging reprinted in: Helgeson MJ, Smith BJ, Johnsen M, et al. Dental considerations for the frail elderly. Spec Care Dent 2002;22:40S–55S.

Table 4
Cardiac risk computation for surgical intervention

Criteria as risk factor	Point index
1. History	
Age ≥ 70 years	5
Myocardial infarction ≤ 6 months	10
2. Physical examination	
S_3 gallop or JVD	11
Valvular aortic stenosis	3
3. Electrocardiogram	
Rhythm other than sinus, PACs On last ECG	7
> 5 PVCs/min documented preoperatively	7
4. General status	
$PO_2 < 60$; $PCO_2 > 50$ mm Hg	
$K < 3.0$, $HCO_3 < 20$ mEq/L	
BUN > 50, Cr > 3.0 mEq/dL	
Abnormal aspartate aminotransferase, chronic liver disease	
Bedridden patients from a noncardiac cause	3
5. Operation	
Intraperitoneal	
Intrathoracic, aortic	3
Emergency	4
Total possible = 53 points	

Adapted from Goldman L, Caldera DL, Nussbaum SR, et al. Multifactorial index of cardiac risk in noncardiac surgical patients. N Eng J Med 1977;297:845–9.

with dyspnea, orthopnea, or pedal edema; recent myocardial infarction [MI]; and syncopal episodes).

Several evidence-based cardiac risk indices then can be applied to stratify patients for noncardiac surgery [44]. Most are predicated on the surgical procedure, specifically, whether or not it is a high-risk, intermediate-risk, or low-risk intervention. Table 4 depicts approximate risk of a major cardiac complication according to Goldman's cardiac risk index. The higher the number of points, the greater the risk of morbidity or mortality [44,45]. Other preoperative assessments include a recent ECG, echocardiograms, consultation with medical colleagues for medications that are being used, and whether or not any antibiotic prophylaxis is indicated prior to surgical intervention. More than half of the cases of bacterial endocarditis that occur in people over age 60 are the result of an increased incidence of cardiac defects and age-related decreased immunocompetence. Most cases of infective endocarditis are not caused by dental treatment, but by dental disease, mastication, and poor oral hygiene [46]. The American Heart Association's protocol 1-hour prior to surgical treatment is well known by practitioners. Adjuvant therapy with 0.12% chlorhexidine rinses is recommended for patients who are susceptible to a bacteremia [47].

The stress of surgical treatment may precipitate serious medical emergencies, such as angina, arrhythmias, MI, stroke, or cardiac arrest. Oral surgeons should be well prepared to apply emergency protocols. If a MI has occurred within a 6-month period, only emergency dental care is undertaken. No elective care should be given to patients who have unstable angina or poorly controlled CHF. Patients who complain of chest pain should be monitored with the ABCs of basic life support. Clothing should be loosened, oxygen should be administered and a 325-mg aspirin can be given except in cases of patients who are sensitive to aspirin, because it can precipitate a bronchospasm. The use of sublingual nitroglycerin (NTG) is warranted in these patients with a dose of 1 tablet every 5 minutes for a total of 3 tablets or until a resolution of symptoms occurs. Patients who have NTG tablets should keep them on the bracket table in case an anginal attack occurs. A blood pressure reading follows each dose, because the vasodilatory effect of NTG can precipitate or exacerbate a significant hypotensive state. Patients also should be questioned about a headache during treatment, because a side effect of NTG is headache. The headache should not be confused with one that can precede the onset of a severe hypertensive episode.

Hypertension

Hypertension is among the most common chronic illnesses seen in the elderly. In patients over age 65, 50% or more have elevations in either their systolic or diastolic pressures that are being treated with antihypertensive medications [48]. All antihypertensive agents should be recorded in the chart and patients reminded to take their doses the morning of surgery. It is prudent to take a blood pressure reading at the first visit in order to have a baseline value prior to surgical procedures, because noticeable fluctuations in blood pressures are seen during anesthetic administration and dental procedures, such as tooth extraction. Proper cuff size is paramount, as many geriatric patients have either a very thin cuff size or an obese cuff size. It is imperative to maintain the cardiovascular reserve of patients and monitor any changes in their hemodynamic status [8]. This may aid in warning of an untoward event and determine the efficacy of their antihypertensive therapy.

A diastolic pressure of 110 mm Hg or greater is contraindicated when elective surgery is considered. Although systolic blood pressure readings have no clear contraindication, the literature suggests a reading greater than 180 mm Hg warrants a postponement of treatment until either medications are re-evaluated or new onset hypertension is diagnosed.

Cardiovascular medications

Anticoagulant therapy

The uses of oral anticoagulants are effective in the management of thromboembolic disorders secondary to cardiovascular insufficiency in the elderly. Possible bleeding diatheses from these medications, however, require careful assessment prior to any surgical therapy. Specific preoperative risk criteria for severe bleeding include patient age and other comorbid illnesses, such as gastrointestinal bleeding, CVA, cardiac arrhythmia, type and chronicity of anemia, and renal disease [20]. Other complications from bleeding include severe capillary fragility, ecchymoses, and necrotic skin lesions that can make access for IV fluids and medications more tenuous [20,49].

Several algorithms exist for the management of patients who are on anticoagulants and require oral surgery. Each decision is based on two criteria: (1) stopping anticoagulant therapy to avoid significant bleeding while (2) not exacerbating the complications of disease for which the anticoagulant is prescribed. Studies show that some patients do not have to discontinue their oral anticoagulant prior to surgery [50]. Other studies suggest that patients discontinue their medication for 72 hours and then resume it the evening or morning after surgery [20,50]. Both studies require that the therapeutic level of anticoagulant is measured by the international normalized ratio (INR). Values at the low end of therapeutic range allow for surgical intervention with a low incidence of severe postoperative bleeding. An INR range of 2.0 to 3.0 for most conditions is acceptable except in patients who have artificial heart valves, which require an INR in the range of 2.5 to 3.5 [47]. A physician consultation should be done to determine patients' current INR level before any procedure that could cause bleeding is done. Usually, when at therapeutic levels, most dentoalveolar procedures can be performed with the use of local hemostatic agents without changing the anticoagulation therapy regimen [50]. For more complicated surgical therapy, inpatient anticoagulation is designed specific to the surgeon's choice (discussed later).

Local hemostatic measures include biting on gauze, sutures, oxidized cellulose, topical thrombin, and tranexamic acid mouthwashes [50]. Many analgesics and antibiotics may affect the level and activity of anticoagulation adversely. Examples of antibiotics that potentiate the action of anticoagulants are dephalosporins, amoxicillin, macrolides, sulpha drugs, and antifungals. Those that diminish anticoagulant activity include rifampin. Anti-inflammatory agents, anticonvulsants, certain antidepressants, and cholesterol-lowering drugs also can exacerbate therapeutic levels of anticoagulants. It is judicious for surgeons to catalogue all medications carefully and determine the risk-to-benefit ratio when prescribing medications that can interact with anticoagulant drugs [20,50].

Other cardiac medications

Patients should maintain their regimens of cardiac medications the day of surgery. Medications commonly prescribed include β-blockers, calcium channel blockers, angiotensin-converting enzyme inhibitors, and centrally acting agents that block α-receptors and β-receptors. It is, however, judicious for surgeons to remember the adverse drug effects of these medications. Antihypertensives, such as α-blockers, β-blockers, calcium channel blockers, and anticholesterol drugs, can cause xerostomia or gingival hyperplasia and precipitate or exacerbate an orthostatic hypotensive episode. In addition, the concomitant use of NSAIDs can antagonize the antihypertensive effects of some medications, whereas opioids may potentiate their hypotensive effects [20]. Table 5 outlines the interactions of antihypertensive agents with pharmacologic agents most commonly prescribed.

Cerebrovascular and neurologic disease

CVA disease is the third leading cause of death in those over 65 years of age. This occurs as a result of a 20% loss of cerebral tissue, a 28% reduction in cerebral blood flow, and a 30% loss in neuron number [48]. Transient ischemic attacks (TIAs), thrombi, emboli, or hemorrhage in the brain further contribute to cerebrovascular disease. Other causes that contribute to CVA are peripheral vascular disease and COPD with thromoboemboli. Risk assessment for neurologic damage is predicated by the symptoms displayed. Individuals who have right brain damage present with a paralyzed left side, spatial perceptual defects, thought impairment, memory deficits, impulsive behavior, and difficulty performing motor tasks, such as oral hygiene. Individuals who have left brain damage may present with a paralyzed right side, language and speech problems, memory deficits, and disorganized behavior.

Table 5
Drug interactions between antihypertensive agents and dental pharmacologic agents

Antihypertensive	Dental agent	Effect	Recommendations
Diuretics			
Furosemide	NSAID	Decreased renal blood flow	Inform about risks versus benefit and consult physician based on stage of hypertension
HCTZ		Loss of antihypertensive effect	
β-adrenergic blockers			
Metoprolol	Epinephrine	Transient hypokalemia	Avoid use if patient is hypokalemic
Atenolol	Levonordefrin NSAID	Decreased renal blood flow	Consult physician based on stage of hypertension
Nonselective β-blockers			
Propanolol	Epinephrine	Hypertension and bradycardia	Monitor blood pressure. Consult physician based on stage of hypertension
Levonordefrin			
Angiotensin-converting enzyme inhibitors			
Captopril	NSAID	Decreased renal blood flow	Consult physician and warn patient
		Loss of antihypertensive effect	Monitor blood pressure
Centrally acting α-adrenergic receptor agonists			
Clonodine	Opioids	Increased central nervous system depression	Use cautiously
		Respiratory depression decreased mental awareness	
Peripheral adrenergic neuronal blockers			
Guanethidine	Epinephrine Levonordephrin	Increased cardiovascular	Use cautiously/monitor blood pressure

Adapted from Yagiela JA, Turner RN. Hypertension. In: Bennett JD, Rosenberg MG, editors. Medical emergencies in dentistry. Philadelphia: WB Saunders; 2002.

Medical consultations should be obtained as needed to assess patients' neurologic status. Patients who have a history of TIAs should be evaluated for carotid stenosis. No elective treatment should be given to patients who have current TIAs or a history of stroke within the prior 6 months. Stress reduction techniques, monitoring of blood pressure, and limits on epinephrine (discussed previously) should be used. Stroke patients also often are on anticoagulation therapy that needs to be managed by the INR (described previously).

Parkinson's disease is seen commonly in the elderly. Movement disorders, such as tremors of the hands, are found in 43% of patients over age 65, which may be attributed either to true Parkinson's or drug-induced Parkinson's. The latter is seen in geriatric patients who are taking calcium channel blockers, methyldopa (Aldomet), haloperidol (Haldol), phenothiazines, and metochlopramide (Reglan) [51]. Drugs that replete endogenous dopamine also may have interactions with the vasoconstrictors in local anesthetics, which compromise cardiovascular function. Again, good documentation of current medicines avoids any undue drug-drug interactions.

Strategies for pain and anxiety management in these patients include inhalation and oral and IV sedation. Specifically, benzodiazepines, opioids, and alkyphenols are good choices. Careful monitoring of blood pressures prevents sudden episodes of hypotension that originate from alterations in autonomic function on smooth muscle from concomitant drug therapy. Pain management strategies are used carefully, because the myocardium becomes more sensitized to vasoconstrictors as a result of the drug therapy for patients who have these neurologic diseases. It is prudent to contact neurologists with any questions about drug-drug interactions.

Respiratory disease

Chronic lower respiratory diseases are the fourth leading cause of death in the elderly [14]. Morphologic changes in pulmonary function associated with aging are decreased elasticity of the chest wall, decreased muscle strength, and decreased vital capacity with less efficient ventilation. Pulmonary diseases in the elderly mainly are of the obstructive airway type (COPD), including chronic bronchitis, emphysema, and adult-onset asthma [52]. The most common perioperative respiratory sequelae are atelectasis, pneumonia, and acute bronchitis. In addition, alterations in esophageal motility can lead to dyspnea and an increased risk for aspiration. The risk for aspiration is much greater in geriatric patients because of diminished protective reflexes and increased gastric emptying time [53]. The latter also can occur in patients who are taking aspirin, NSAIDs, and β-adrenergic blockers, such as those in ophthalmic solutions used for glaucoma. Accumulation of aspirates then sets the stage for pneumonia and prolonged hospitalizations that can cripple healthy and unhealthy geriatric patients.

Patients who have pulmonary problems may require appointments scheduled during the late morning or the afternoon to allow for a period of readjustment to clear their lungs of fluid that accumulates from being supine at night. Patient positioning during treatment should be either upright or no greater than a 45° angle. This allows for easy access and ability to breathe without restriction. Many patients who have COPD can suffer from syncopal episodes secondary to continuous coughing with diminished venous return and concomitant reflex vasodilatation. Even the mildest of sedation strategies and surgical procedures can result in hypoventilation with concomitant atelectasis and increase the risk for hypoxemia and infection during the postsurgical period. The administration of oxygen requires careful titration, because patients who have COPD disease require a continuous hypoxic drive. The dosing is low flow of 2 liters per minute versus the normal use of 4 liters of oxygen through a nasal cannula. Patients who are on long-term corticosteroids may require loading doses to avoid stress-induced adrenal suppression when surgical treatment is scheduled. The additional problems of xerostomia from certain medications and palatal necrosis from the use of corticosteroid inhalers make treatment decisions complex. It is judicious to check with the patient's physician as to whether or not pulmonary function testing is necessary prior to any surgical procedure.

Perioperative precautions for patients who have pulmonary disease include increased use of bronchodilators, encourage coughing, deep breathing incentive spirometry, and mobility [54]. Nitrous oxide and oxygen sedation may be considered based on the type of respiratory problem. If patients develop dyspnea during treatment, dentists need to consider cause: pulmonary, psychologic, cardiovascular, allergic, foreign body, and so forth. Patients are assessed with auscultation and respiratory rate to determine if any obstruction is present resulting from foreign bodies or secretions. It is judicious for practitioners to have an emergency drug kit in their practice that contains β-agonist bronchodilators. The onset of action occurs within a few minutes and doses can be repeated for several rounds. Treatment then should be discontinued and patients rescheduled with possible medical reassessment before further treatment.

Smoking and pulmonary complications

Smoking cessation is pivotal in reducing the risks of pulmonary complications. Prospective studies suggest improved postoperative complication rates in patients who stop smoking for up to 2 months prior to surgery [55]. Perioperative strategies consist of discontinued tobacco use for a minimum of 2 to 3 weeks to allow for decreased hypersecretion of mucus and tracheobronchial clearance that compromise their postoperative course. Although there is no evidence-based data for a specific algorithm, postoperative treatment for patients who are smokers include chest physiotherapy, incentive spirometry, bronchodilators, steroids, and empiric antibiotic therapy as needed [55,56].

Thomboembolic complications

Thromboembolic complications during the perioperative period are a common event. Studies suggest that 20% to 30% of patients undergoing surgical interventions without prophylaxis are predisposed to developing pulmonary emboli secondary to deep vein thrombosis [56–58]. The incidence rate of deep venous thrombosis increases with age and accounts for a large proportion of operative complications in elderly persons as a result of compromise of respiratory and cardiovascular function [53]. Management strategies to avoid the occurrence of thromboembolic events include clinical examination and preoperative imaging. The gold standard for diagnosis of pulmonary emboli is the ventilation-perfusion scan [58]. Suggestions for prophylaxis against thromboembolic events include the use of low molecular weight heparin or adjusted-dose warfarin with an INR maintained in the 2 to 3 range [57,58]. Perioperative measures suggested most often are 5000 U subcutaneous heparin 6 to 8 hours before surgery and then 8 to 12 hours during the postoperative period for up to 7 days [57]. The choices for anticoagulation, however, must be monitored carefully to avoid catastrophic hemorrhagic events that can hamper even the most routine of surgical procedures. Aspirin, intermittent pneumatic devices, compression stockings and early postoperative ambulation are advantageous for all elderly patients during the perioperative and postoperative period in order to decrease the risk for deep venous thrombosis and pulmonary emboli.

Endocrine disorders

Diabetes mellitus

Diabetes mellitus (DM) is a common illness in the geriatric population, affecting more than 20% who are age 65 or older [59]. Adult onset non–insulin-dependent DM (type 2 DM) is the most common form encountered. DM is a clinical predictor of perioperative myocardial ischemia because of the association between DM and coronary artery disease and the increased incidence of other perioperative complications, including stroke, renal failure, diabetic ketoacidosis, and sepsis. Elevated blood glucose levels (greater than 300 mg/dL) set the stage for increased infection resulting from poor wound healing [8,60]. In addition, hyperglycemia causes an increased red blood cell turgor and viscosity and decreased polymorphonuclear leukocyte chemotactic mechanisms. The latter hampers cellular defenses. Concomitant impairment of healing coupled with cardiovascular, renal, and neurologic impairment ultimately compromise successful surgical outcomes.

Diabetics are most commonly referred to oral surgery practitioners because of their prevalence of oral-health related sequelae (ie, severe odontogenic abscesses, xerostomia, burning mouth, and fungal infections) [61]. It is important to assess diabetic patients' level of glycemic control prior to surgical intervention. Patients should be asked about their glucose levels, frequency of testing levels, and compliance with diabetic medications. Scheduling of appointments for diabetic patients is predicated on their level of glycemic control. Patients who have type 2 DM that is well controlled with diet and exercise require no alteration in the perioperative treatment plan. Those patients who require hypoglycemic agents should take their medications the night before or discontinue them for up to 2 to 3 days prior to surgery (based on the half-life of the agent), resuming it that evening depending on their blood glucose level [61,62]. A common complication that can occur in elderly diabetics is a hypoglycemic episode. Before an appointment is started, patients should be asked when their last meal was and their most recent blood glucose level. An acceptable target range for blood glucose is 150 to 200 mg/dL. Patients on oral hypoglycemic agents should hold their medication the day of surgery and treat hyperglycemia with short-acting insulin until they can resume the oral agents. It is imperative for surgeons to remember that oral hypoglycemics as a drug group can contribute to bouts of leukopenia and thrombocytopenia that can exacerbate wound infections, severe bleeding, and delayed wound healing

[20,61,62]. The early identification and rapid treatment of a hypoglycemic episode avoids more serious complications of seizures and coma (Box 3) [62].

Guidelines for self-monitoring blood glucose levels are straightforward in patients who have insulin-dependent DM (type 1 DM). The American Dental Association currently recommends evaluation of the level of glycosylated hemoglobin (range $\leq 7.0\%$), which reflects the mean level of glycemic control for a period of 2 to 3 months. This assay is shown to be a predictor of development of postoperative complications [61]. The hyperglycemic state is easier to treat than hypoglycemic episode. Patients who type 1 DM and have single-dose per day insulin are advised to reduce dosing of insulin to 50% to 66% the morning of surgery; IV fluids are administered with glucose. Patients who need multiple dosing of insulin receive 50% preoperatively with glucose solutions followed by a sliding-scale insulin regimen as needed [61,62]. Extensive procedures requiring hospital admission and a nothing-by-mouth status require a prior medical clearance in order to readjust medication dosing and nutritional requirements. Monitoring blood glucose levels before and during the surgical procedure is accomplished with a sliding-scale regimen of regular insulin. This is continued in order to readjust any dosing of their medications. Blood glucose monitoring is predicated on duration of therapy and the degree of metabolic control to be achieved.

Antibiotic therapy is recommended in all surgical patients who have diabetes because of increased risk for infection and poor wound healing. The dosages may need to be reduced in the elderly because of the compromised renal and hepatic function seen most often as a result of diabetes [62]. Elderly patients are especially susceptible to unusual infections, such as malignant external otitis, necrotizing fasciitis, and rhinocerebral mucormycosis. Empiric antibiotic treatment therapies that decrease the degree of oral disease after extensive surgical procedures concomitantly decrease the risks for further multiorgan failure.

Thyroid disease

Many thyroid disorders occur with advancing age because of age-related changes in the morphology and physiology of the gland [63]. Subclinical hyperthyroidism and hypothyroidism thus are seen frequently in the geriatric population. Unlike younger populations, elderly patients often have multiple complex illnesses with their thyroid disease, including osteoporosis, DM, lipid abnormalities, autoimmune diseases, dementia, and malnutrition, that tend to exacerbate the subclinical manifestations of thyroid dysfunction [64]. In addition, geriatric patients who have unexplained atrial fibrillation and high-output cardiac failure with angina may be diagnosed with a hyperthyroid state, referred to as thyrotoxicosis. Most of the elderly also can develop hypothyroidism secondary to an autoimmune thyroiditis [65]. A detailed medical history should elicit clues suggestive of either a hyperthyroid state or a hypothyroid condition, because hypothyroid patients may be euthyroid at the present time with medications. Assessment of thyroid medications allows surgeons to tailor specific anesthetic and pain management strategies for patients. Hormonal replacement therapy for geriatric patients versus younger patients varies considerably. Young patients who have hypothyroidism usually take 75 to 150 μg synthroid per day, whereas geriatric patients are titrated at 25 μg per day to prevent coronary occlusion and angina. Patients may record allergies to vasoconstrictors, caffeine, and cola if they are hyperthyroid and central nervous system depressants, benzodiazepines, and antihistamines if they are hypothyroid [64,66].

Elective and emergent surgical intervention requires careful evaluation of thyroid function. Severe hypothyroidism and hyperthyroidism (thyroid storm) are associated with significant increases in perioperative morbidity and mortality. Untreated hypothyroidism can exacerbate depression and respiratory insufficiency and slow down drug metabolism. Complications of hyperthyroidism of surgical significance are fever, tachyarrhthmias, and CHF [66]. Within an office setting, the treatment of patients who have thyroid problems is based on symptomatology. Until a definitive diagnosis is established, all elective surgical therapy should be avoided with only palliative treatment rendered. Elective procedures

---

Box 3. Risk factors for a hypoglycemic episode in the elderly

Sulfonylurea or insulin therapy
Renal insufficiency
Liver disease
Cognitive impairment
Autonomic neuropathy
Malnutrition
ETOH
Sedative agents
Polypharmacy
Recent hospitalization
Cardiovascular disease

can be done on patients who are euthyroid. In cases of emergent surgery, medical clearance of hypothyroid patients involves dosing with corticosteroids and levothyroxine. In patients who have hyperthyroidism who require emergent surgical intervention, patients' endocrinologists can prescribe propylthiouracil, corticosteroids, and β-blockers. An acute exacerbation of patients who have a hyperthyroid state can lead to a thyrotoxic crisis, or thyroid storm, often seen in hyperthyroid patients who are poorly treated and who have undergone sudden increases in stress, sepsis, or emergency surgery. A physical examination reveals fever, palpitations, and tachycardia. Blood pressure monitoring reveals a hypotensive state and if an ECG is placed, patients may exhibit cardiac arrhythmias. All treatment is stopped and patients are given oxygen. Access for an intravenous line should be attempted and patients then given IV fluids depending on their other medical problems (dextrose in normal saline versus lactated ringers, depending on other systemic illnesses). The use of NTG tablets is not contraindicated but monitoring of blood pressure is imperative to avoid significant hypotension (discussed previously). An established office algorithm for endocrine emergencies should be in place with staff drills.

Arthritis

Arthritis is the most common chronic disease in adults, with 38% afflicted at ages older than 65 years [43]. Its affect on muscles, bones, and ligaments cause many to suffer during the most simple daily routines. Patients who have arthritis are prescribed many medications containing aspirin, NSAIDs, and corticosteroids that may cause or exacerbate severe bleeding, wound healing, and ulcerations that complicate surgical therapy. A recent update of prescribed medicines allows for readjustments and bolus steroid dosing depending on the invasiveness of the procedure.

Antibiotic prophylaxis often is considered on an individual basis. Although the risk for prosthetic joint infection is low (0.5%–5.0%), it is a major cause of joint failure. The advisory committee jointly developed by the American Academy of Orthopedic Surgeons and the American Dental Association has a consensus statement as to recommendations for antibiotic prophylaxis in patients who have joint replacements: "Antibiotic prophylaxis is not indicated for dental patients with pins, plates, screws, nor is it routinely indicated for most dental patients with total joint replacements. However it is advisable to consider premedication in a small number of patients who may be at potential increased risk for hematogenous total joint infection" [67]. Antibiotic prophylaxis is suggested within the first 2 years after joint replacement, if there was previous joint infection, and in patients who have immunosuppression, inflammatory arthropathies, and type 1 DM, because bacteremias can cause hematogenous spread.

Oral surgeons should provide an environment that minimizes these symptoms. Positioning in the dental chair and use of neck pillows and special cushions can make the treatment comfortable. Issues of postoperative care may involve homecare with special irrigation and ergonomic adjustments as advised by their physical therapists. It also is judicious for surgeons to stress that the use of OTC medications can cause adverse events when used with postoperative drugs (discussed previously).

Dementia and postoperative delirium

Cognitive dysfunction in elderly surgical patients can present as either dementia or delirium. Dementia is a syndrome characterized by deterioration of the organic functions of the brain that is chronic and usually lasting more than 1 year. The risk of dementia increases 0.01% to 0.74% in age 60 and over per year, with 2.2% to 3.5% per year over age 80 [68]. Symptoms of delirium may mimic those of dementia. Delirium, however, has a rapid onset and is characterized by a fluctuating state of alertness, confusion, disorientation, memory impairment, apprehension, and agitation. More than 15% of elderly patients who undergo surgery are susceptible to some form of postoperative delirium [69]. The most common cause of delirium stems from drug toxicity and metabolic problems. Other causes of delirium are malnutrition, dehydration, uncontrolled endocrine disorders, organ failure, stress of surgery, and length of the operation [68]. As such, delirium is a more acute, usually reversible disorder secondary to a concomitant medical problem.

Surgeons should be cognizant of the timeline when the symptoms of delirium first occur. Studies indicate a period of 4 days with a prodromal phase. Subtle behavioral changes are noted during the immediate postoperative period and become erratic as the delirium progresses. Patients can present initially as depressed, perplexed, or agitated [70]. The treatment strategies for postoperative delirium include rapid laboratory panels of liver function, urinalysis, complete blood count, serum urea nitrogen (SUN), creatinine, drug screens for therapeutic ranges and determinations of toxic levels of drugs. CT is essential to rule out bleeding diatheses and presence of fluid indicative of any brain infection. Spinal taps also are indicated, especially in patients who have comorbid illnesses, such as diabetes and thromboemboli. Careful monitoring of fluid and electrolytes is imperative to avoid neurologic sequelae of hypernatremia, hyponatremia, and surgically induced diabetes insipidus. The use of certain anesthetic drugs with anticholinergic properties should be documented, because a strong correlation exists between this drug and mental dysfunction [56].

Recommendations exist for the use of a short-acting anxiolytic to control agitation, combativeness, and possible hallucinations. Again, the risk-to-benefit ratio must be considered with respect to strength of sedation versus respiratory depression, because the latter can exacerbate the degree of confusion already present. Family support also may be good medicine, because caregivers can help reorient these patients to person, place, and time. Familiar objects can be used as reminders of the preoperative period. Most cases of postoperative delirium resolve in 1 to 2 weeks as the underlying cause is corrected. Cases that remain unchanged over a few months are associated with increased morbidity and mortality as a result of postoperative complications that increase length of hospital stay.

Summary and conclusions

Oral and maxillofacial surgeons will be treating a significantly greater number of geriatric patients, especially with the aging of the baby boomer generation. As such, there will be a concomitant need not only for high quality surgical care but also a more global approach for total health care. Suggested criteria for optimal surgical outcome in the elderly are:

- Never use age as the sole criterion for surgery.
- Assess comorbid medical conditions and stabilize during the preoperative period.
- Review all medications preoperatively, including OTC medications, to avoid adverse drug effects.
- Determine cognitive ability and ability to undergo informed consent.
- Consider noninvasive assessment of cardiac status for all geriatric patients, regardless of risk.
- Monitor patients preoperatively for nutritional and fluid and electrolyte deficits.
- Prophylaxis is imperative for risk of thromboembolism and endocarditis.
- Ask about pain often; use individually scheduled or patient-controlled analgesic dosing.
- Mobilize promptly and control pain on an individual basis.
- Monitor risk for postoperative delirium.

References

[1] National Center for Health Statistics. Vital statistics of the United States. 1984. Public Health Service. DHHS publications Washington, DC: Government Printing Office; 1987. p. 87–122. Available at: http://www.agingstats.gov/chartbook2004/ordercopy.html.

[2] Berg R, Morgenstern NE. Physiologic changes in the elderly. Dent Clin North Am 1997;41:651–68.

[3] Vaz FG, Seymour DG. A prospective study of elderly general surgical patients: preoperative medical problems. Age Ageing 1989;18:309–15.

[4] Dunlop WE, Rosenblood L, Lawrence L, et al. Effects of age and severity of illness on outcome and length of stay in geriatric surgical patients. Am J Surg 1993; 165:577–80.

[5] Berkey DB, Ettinger RL. Assessment of the older adult. In: Papas AS, Niessen LC, Chauncy HH, editors. Geriatric dentistry: aging and oral health. St. Louis: Mosby Year Book; 1991.

[6] Levy SM, Jakobsen JR. A comparison of medical histories reported by dental patients and their physicians. Special Care Dent 1991;11:26–31.

[7] Wolinsky FD, Pendergaast JM, Miller DK, et al. A preliminary validation of a nutritional risk measure for the elderly. Prev Med 1985;1:53–9.

[8] Tully CL. Medical evaluation of the aging patient. Oral Maxillofac Clin North Am 1996;8:171–85.

[9] Sullivan DW, Walls RC, Lipshitz DA. Protein energy, under nutrition and the risk of mortality within one year of hospital discharge in a select population of geriatric rehabilitation patients. Am J Clin Nutr 1991; 53:599–605.

[10] Boosalis MG, Stiles NJ. Nutritional needs of the elderly. Oral Maxillofac Clin North Am 1996;8:199–206.

[11] Luckey AE, Parsa CJ. Fluids and electrolytes in the aged. Arch Surg 2003;38:1055–60.

[12] Warner MA, Offord KP, Warner ME, et al. Role of preoperative cessation of smoking and other factors in postoperative pulmonary complications: a blinded prospective study of CABG patients. Mayo Clin Proc 1989;64:609–16.

[13] Thomas VS, Rockwood KJ. Alcohol abuse, cognitive impairment, and mortality among older people. J Am Geriatr Soc 2001;49:415–20.

[14] Kilmartin CM. Managing the medically compromised geriatric patient. J Prosthet Dent 1994;72:492–9.

[15] Blazer D. Techniques for communicating with your elderly patient. Geriatrics 1978;33:79–84.

[16] Michocki RJ, Laing PP, Hooper FJ, et al. Drug prescribing for the elderly. Arch Fam Med 1993;2:441–4.

[17] Melamed SF. Anxiety and pain control in the older patient. Spec Care Dent 1987;7:22–3.

[18] Greenblatt DJ, Seller EM, Shader RS. Drug therapy: drug disposition in old age. N Engl J Med 1982;306: 1081–8.
[19] Smallman JM, Powell H, Ewart MC, et al. Ketrolac for postoperative analgesia in elderly patients. Anesthesia 1992;47:149–52.
[20] Davis GA, Chandler MH. Drug therapy and drug interactions. Oral Maxillofac Clin North Am 1996;8:245–63.
[21] Wilder-Smith CH, Schinke J, Osterwalder J, et al. Oral Tramadol: a mucopoid agonist and monoamine re-uptake-blocker and morphine for strong cancer-related pain. Ann Oncol 1994;5:141–6.
[22] Rauck RL, Ruoff GE, McMillen JI. comparison of tramadol and acetamenophen with codeine for long-term pain management in elderly patients. Curr Ther Res 1994;55:1417–21.
[23] Quinn CL. The physically compromised patient. In: Malamed SF, editor. Sedation: a guide to patient management. 3rd edition. St. Louis: Mosby; 1985. p. 609–17.
[24] Ryder W, Wright PA. Dental sedation. A review. Br Dent J 1988;165:207–16.
[25] Dionne RA, Yagiela JA, Moore PA, et al. Comparing efficacy and safety of four intravenous sedation regimens in dental outpatients. J Am Dent Assoc 2001;132: 740–51.
[26] Ghezzi EM, Chavez EM, Ship JA. General anesthesia protocol for the dental patient: emphasis for older patients. Special Care Dent 2000;20:81–93.
[27] Helgeson MJ, Smith BJ, Johnsen M, et al. Dental considerations for the frail elderly. Spec Care Dent 2002;22:40S–55S.
[28] Hollonsten AL, Koch G, Schroder U. Nitrous oxide—oxygen sedation in dental care. Commun Dent Oral Epidemiol 1983;11:347–55.
[29] Holzman RS, Cullen DJ, Eichhorn JH, et al. Guidelines for sedation by non-anesthesiologists during diagnosis and therapeutic procedures. J Clin Anesth 1994;6:265–76.
[30] Matear DW, Clarke D. Considerations for the use of oral sedation in the institutionalized geriatric patient during dental interventions: a review of the literature. Spec Care Dent 1999;19:56–63.
[31] Buxbaum JL, Schwartz AJ. Perianesthetic considerations for the elderly patient. Surg Clin North Am 1994;74:41–58.
[32] Loeffler PM. Oral benzodiazepines and conscious sedation : a review. J Oral Maxillofac Surg 1992;50: 989–97.
[33] Galli MT, Henry RG. Using intravenous sedation to manage adults with neurological impairment. Spec Care Dent 1999;19:275–80.
[34] Campbell RL, Smith PB. Intravenous sedation in 200 geriatric patients undergoing office surgery. Anesth Prog 1997;44:64–7.
[35] Muravchick S. The elderly outpatient: current anesthetic implications. Curr Opin Anaesthesiol 2002;15: 621–5.
[36] Kitagawa E, Iida A, Kimura Y, et al. Responses to intravenous sedation by elderly patients at the Hokkaido University Dental Hospital. Anesth Prog 1992; 39:73–88.
[37] Ineke Neutel C, Hirdes JP, Maxwell CJ, et al. New evidence on benzodiazepine use and falls: the time factor. Age Ageing 1996;25:273–8.
[38] Tiret L, Desmonts JM, Hatton F, et al. Complications associated with anesthesia: a prospective survey in France. Can Anesth Soc J 1986;33:336–44.
[39] Hosking MP, Warner MA, Lobdell CM, et al. Outcomes of surgery in patients 90 years of age and older. JAMA 1989;261:1909–15.
[40] Muravchick S. Anesthesia for the elderly. In: Miller RD, editor. Anesthesia. 4th ed. New York: Churchhill-Livingston; 1994. p. 2143–56.
[41] Pedersen T, Eliasen K, Henriksen E. A prospective study of risk factors and cardiopulmonary complications associated with anesthesia and surgery: risk indicators of cardiopulmonary morbidity. Acta Anaesthesiol Scand 1990;34:144–55.
[42] Bennett JA, Lingaraja N, Horrow JC, et al. Elderly patients recover more rapidly from Desflurane than Isoflurane anesthesia. J Clin Anesth 1992;4:378–81.
[43] Berg W, Morgenstern NE. Physiologic changes in the elderly. Dent Clin North Am 1998;41:651–68.
[44] Goldman L. Cardiac risk in non-cardiac surgery: an update. Anesth Analg 1995;80:810–20.
[45] Goldman L. Assessment of perioperative cardiac risk. N Engl J Med 1994;297:845–50.
[46] Thomas DR, Ritchie CS. Preoperative assessment of older adults. J Am Geriatr Soc 1995;43:811–21.
[47] Rose LF, Mealey B, Minsk L, et al. Oral care for patients with cardiovascular disease and stroke. J Am Dent Assoc 2002;133:375–82.
[48] Petito AR, Carlotti AE. Cerebrovascular accident (stroke). In: Bennett JD, Rosenberg MB, editors. Medical emergencies in dentistry. Philadelphia: WB Saunders; 2002. p. 213–28.
[49] Beyth RJ, Landefeld CS. Anticoagulants in older patients: a safety perspective. Drugs Aging 1995;6:45–50.
[50] Dodson TB. Strategies for managing anticoagulated patients requiring dental extractions: an exercise in evidence-based clinical practice. J Mass Dent Soc 2002;501:44–50.
[51] Gelb DJ, Oliver E, Gilman S. Diagnostic criteria for Parkinson disease. Arch Neurol 1999;56:33–9.
[52] Seymour DG. Respiratory system in the elderly surgical patient. In: Medical Assessment of the elderly surgical patient. London: Croom Helm; 1986. p. 24–77.
[53] Brooks-Brunn JA. Validation of a predictor model for postoperative pulmonary complications. Heart Lung 1998;27:151–6.
[54] Byrd RB. Preventing pulmonary complications of surgery. Respir Ther 1982;12:37–42.
[55] Warner MA, Tinker JH, Divertie MB. Pre-operative cessation of smoking and pulmonary complications in pulmonary dysfunction. Anesthesiology 1983;59:A60.
[56] Synan WJ. Postoperative management and complication. Oral Maxillofac Clin North Am 1996;8:265–80.

[57] Hirsh J. Pulmonary embolism in the elderly. Cardiol Clin 1991;9:457–74.
[58] Thomas DR, Ritchie CS. Perioperative assessment of older adults. J Am Geriatr Soc 1995;43:811–21.
[59] Sarasin DS, Westlund KJ. Diabetes mellitus. In: Bennett JD, Rosenberg MB, editors. Medical emergencies in dentistry. Philadelphia: WB Saunders; 2002. p. 141–52.
[60] Miloro M, McCormick S. Wound healing and immunity. Oral Maxillofac Clin North Am 1996;8:159–70.
[61] Lalla RV, D'Ambrosio JA. Dental management considerations for the patient with diabetes mellitus. J Am Dent Assoc 2001;132:1425–32.
[62] Danese RD, Aron DC. Diabetes in the elderly. In: Landefeld CS, Palmer RM, Johnson MA, editors. Current geriatric diagnosis and treatment. New York: Lange Medical Books/McGraw Hill; 2004. p. 338–47.
[63] Halpern LR, Chase DCC. Perioperative management of patients with endocrine dysfunction. Oral Maxillofac Surg Clin NA 1998;10:491–500.
[64] Shetty KR, Duthie EH. Thyroid disease and associated illness in the elderly. Clin Geriatr Med 1995;11: 311–25.
[65] Gilbert PL. Preoperative evaluation of the patient with endocrine disease. Mt Sinai J Med 1991;58:8–68.
[66] Federman DD. Hyperthyroidism in the geriatric population. Hosp Pract 1991;26:61–70.
[67] Advisory Statement of American Academy of Orthopedic Surgeons and American Dental Association on Antibiotic Prophylaxis for Dental Patients with total Joint Replacements. AAOS Bull 1997;45(3). Available at: http://www.aaos.org/wordhtml/papers/advistmt/1014.htm.
[68] O'Keeffe ST, Chonchubhair AN. Postoperative delirium in the elderly. Br J Anaesth 1994;73:673–87.
[69] Millar HR. Psychiatric morbidity in elderly surgical patients. Br J Psychol 1981;138:17–20.
[70] Williams MA, Campbell EB, Raynor WJ, et al. Reducing acute confusional states in elderly patients with hip fractures. Res Nurs Health 1985;8:329–37.

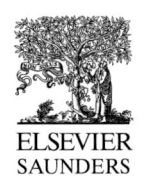

Perioperative Considerations in the Management of Pediatric Surgical Patients

Mark J. Steinberg, DDS, MD*, Andrés F. Herrera, DDS

Division of Oral and Maxillofacial Surgery and Dental Medicine, Loyola Stritch School of Medicine, Loyola University Medical Center, 2160 South First Avenue, Maywood, IL 60153, USA

Most lectures and articles concerning pediatric management usually start out by pointing out that children are not little adults. This certainly is true and is the reason to include a separate discussion of pediatric management. Pediatric anatomy and physiology differ significantly from those of adults and, therefore, require special considerations in evaluation and perioperative management. This article highlights the anatomic and physiologic differences that influence pediatric management. It also covers specific disease processes that are common in the pediatric population and may involve special management strategies.

In recent years, there has been an increased focus by public media concerning the attention provided to children by health care practitioners [1]. Further scrutiny has been placed on dentistry as a result of various cases of adverse outcomes involving children in the dental setting. In 2000, Cote and colleagues [2] reported 95 cases of adverse outcomes involving sedation. They found 51 deaths and 9 cases of permanent neurologic injury. Dentistry was the specialty most highly associated with adverse events, accounting for 33% of them. Among the dental specialties, oral and maxillofacial surgeons were involved in 34% of these cases. Drug interactions and inadequate resuscitation were the most common factors associated with poor outcomes. The fifth most common factor of the 95 cases was inappropriate preoperative evaluation. The same investigators, in the same year [3], analyzed the same 95 adverse events in relation to the medications used during sedation. They found that the use of three or more medications in combination was associated significantly with the development of poor outcomes. The addition of nitrous oxide to other medications in a nonhospital-based setting was the most commonly observed pattern associated with poor results. Both of these findings were associated with procedures performed in the dental setting.

Anatomy and physiology

A thorough understanding of pediatric anatomy and physiology are essential when planning any treatment of this particular patient population.

In any procedure in the oral and maxillofacial region, the airway is involved by direct manipulation within its boundaries and by indirect effect of anesthetic techniques. The head in pediatric patients accounts for a much larger percentage of the body size compared with an adult's head. At the same time, the external occipital eminence is more prominent and the neck is shorter. These characteristics make the pediatric airway prone to obstruction, especially when patients are in a reclined or seated position. In general, the pediatric airway is smaller compared with the adult airway. At the same time, the tongue size is proportionally larger than the mandible; this structure is positioned more superiorly, as the larynx is located more rostrally. Special consideration should be made for children during mixed dentition. The presence of loose, ready-to-exfoliate primary teeth is

---

* Corresponding author.
 E-mail address: msteinb@lumc.edu (M.J. Steinberg).

a potential risk for aspiration and should be handled carefully.

Hypertrophy of the lymphoid tissue at the level of tonsils and adenoids, common in this patient population, decreases the overall airway space further. For preoperative evaluation and medicolegal documentation, it always is appropriate to classify the airway and the tonsillar hypertrophy. Mallampati and colleagues' [4] airway classification is the most widely used. Four types of airways are identified based on the visibility of the uvula, soft palate, and oropharyngeal structures with the mouth open on an upright position (Fig. 1). Brodsky and colleagues, in 1987 [5], outlined a tonsillar hypertrophy classification according to the percentage of airway obstruction. Type 0 includes tonsils within the palatine fossa, not causing any airway obstruction. In type 1 +, there is a 25% obstruction of the airway; type 2 +, the obstruction is 25% to 50%; type 3 +, airway obstruction of 50% to 75%; and type 4 + more than 75% airway obstruction. In 1997, Fishbaugh and coworkers [6] demonstrated the relationship between tonsillar hypertrophy and airway obstruction during sedation. They found that 83% of the patients who had enlarged tonsils developed apnea during the procedure. In addition, 100% of the patients who had tonsillar hypertrophy evidenced significant oxygen desaturation during sedation. Tonsillar and adenoid hypertrophy account for the most common cause of sleep apnea and its comorbidities in pediatric patients [7,8] versus adult patients, in whom sleep apnea is greatly associated with obesity. Cardiac abnormalities often are associated with obstructive sleep apnea, including hypertrophy of the right or left ventricle [9]. Obesity may or may not play a role in the development of pediatric sleep apnea. Careful attention should be paid to parents reporting patients who have history of snoring, presence of enlarged or pharyngeal lymphoid tissue, and elevated body mass index (BMI), as they may be at increased risk for sleep-disordered breathing (SDB) and obstructive sleep apnea [10,11]. In addition, Gozal and Burnside, in 2004 [12], demonstrated that the upper airway collapsibility increases in children who have obstructive sleep apnea after the application of topical anesthesia. They propose that the maintenance of a patent airway during wakefulness in children who have SDB requires tonic activation of topical mechanisms that induce the activation of the upper dilator muscles. In conclusion, SDB and obstructive sleep apnea can be potentiated pharmacologically by the use of sedative medications and topical anesthetics used routinely in the oral and maxillofacial surgery setting.

As discussed previously, the larynx is positioned more rostrally and superiorly. The narrowest point of the airway, in children, is not at the vocal cords but at the criocoid cartilage. This characteristic precludes the use of cuffed endotracheal tubes in children younger than 6 years of age.

The pediatric airway, compared with the adult, is smaller in diameter throughout its extension. The number of gas-exchanging units at birth is 20 million per lung. This number increases to 300 million mature alveoli by 8 years of age [13]. As a result of this characteristic, the airway resistance in pediatric patients is higher than in adults. According to Poiseuille's law, $\Delta P = V8\eta L/\pi r^4$ (where ΔP is airway resistance, η is viscosity, L is tube length, and r is radius of the tube), the airway resistance is directly proportional to the length of the conducting tube and inversely proportional to its radius at the fourth power. Based on this law, any decrease in the airway diameter as a result of secretions and wall inflammation, as seen in asthma and upper respiratory infection (URI), has a significant adverse effect on the airway resistance and, finally, on the gas exchange process [13]. The ventilatory mechanics in pediatric patients also is affected adversely by the presence of immature accessory muscles of respiration and by a more horizontal configuration of the ribs. Thus, pediatric patients depend more on diaphragmatic breathing for their ventilatory requirements. In terms

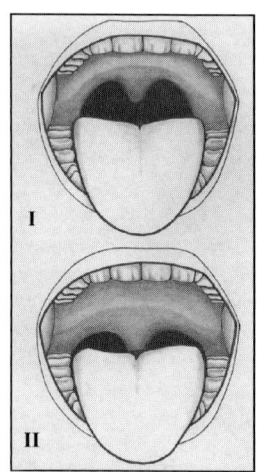

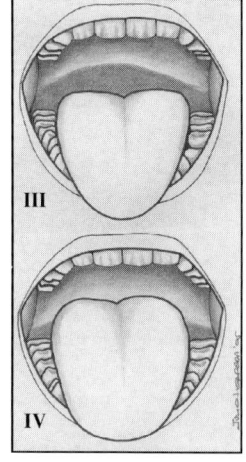

Fig. 1. Mallampati's upper airway classification based on the size of the tongue and visualization of the pharyngeal structures on mouth opening. Class I: soft palate, anterior and posterior tonsillar pillars, and uvula are visible. Class II: anterior and posterior tonsillar pillars and tip of the ulula are obscured by the base of the tongue. Class III: only the soft palate is visible. Class IV: soft palate is not visible.

of lung volumes, the pediatric functional residual capacity is lower because of the lack of elastin on the airways. A lower functional residual capacity means a more rapid oxygen desaturation in the presence of airway obstruction.

Cardiac output (CO) is determined by the heart rate and the stroke volume. The stroke volume is determined by the preload, contractility, and the afterload. Up to age 2, the CO depends mainly on changes of the heart rate. Other factors affecting the CO in infant patients are less effective than in children and adults. The preload is dependent on the myocardial fiber stretch at the end of diastole. The immature heart of infants is less compliant and, therefore, increases of end-diastolic pressure are not translated as equal increases on the end-diastolic volume and fiber length. Lower concentration of contractile fibers and the presence of underdeveloped sarcoplasmic reticulum affect the contractility properties of the neonate heart negatively. There also is an autonomic imbalance of the infant cardiovascular system. The sympathetic nervous system is underdeveloped and for that reason the heart is under higher parasympathetic control and stimulation. Sinus bradycardia is the most common response to a variety of conditions, including hypoxia and hypercarbia [13].

After birth, the development and maturation of the gastrointestinal system continues, increasing the length of the intestine and the total absorptive surface area, the latter at the expense of the maturation of the villous architecture and the formation of plicae circulares [13]. Table 1 outlines the significant gastrointestinal factors through different growth stages, which can affect the absorption of medications given orally. Hepatic function also continues its maturation after gestational life. Hepatic function reaches adult levels by late childhood. In the neonate, liver function is altered by a decreased functional capacity of the hepatocyte. Protein production, metabolism, and clearance of substances and medications all are affected during this phase. Abnormal glycogen and biliurrubin metabolism and biotransformation of liver metabolized drugs also are affected and should be taken into consideration when planning any surgical procedures or prescribing medications. Longer duration of action should be expected for medications with high protein bindin, such as local anesthetics and sedative medications.

The percentage of total body water at term birth is 78%. This value is significantly higher in adults. This percentage decreases slowly over the first 2 years of age to 60% of total body weight. This characteristic may influence higher dosages of water-soluble medications, such as many antibiotics. Alternatively, lower subcutaneous fat content and lean body mass in infants and children may affect the pharmacokinetics of lipid-soluble medications in which redistribution is the main mechanism for termination of their effect. Longer duration of action should be expected when using these types of medication in this patient population [14].

Mature renal function is reached by 2 years of age. During the first 2 years, however, glomerular filtration and tubular excretion and reabsorption are significantly lower than adult values. Neonatal glomerular filtration is 25% of adult values and the maximum urine concentration of infants reaches only 500 to 600 mOsm/kg versus 1200 mOsm/kg in adults. These factors are associated with poor tolerance to dehydration and water overload in infants.

Temperature monitoring and control are essential in pediatric patients, especially during the first 2 years of life. Larger body surface area (BSA), decreased lean body mass, and subcutaneous fat account for the crucial differences in temperature regulation in infant patients compared with children or adults. Heat loss in infants mainly is a consequence of radiation, convection, and evaporation [15].

The energy requirements of pediatric patients are significantly higher than those of adult patients. These higher energy demands are a consequence of a higher basal metabolic rate (BMR) and satisfy the caloric needs involved in growth. Energy requirement levels decrease with age, equaling adult needs once physical growth has stopped.

An estimated BMR for term neonates is 45 to 50 kcal/kg/d compared with a BMR of 20 to 25 kcal/kg/d in adults. Lower caloric demands are seen in children who have an estimated BMR of 30 to 35 kcal/kg/d. Higher energy demands are to be expected in postsurgical, trauma and burned patients [13].

Table 1
Physiologic factors that influence the oral absorption of medications

Parameter	Neonate	Infant	Child
Gastric acid secretion	Reduced	Normal	Normal
Gastric emptying time	Decreased	Increased	Increased
Intestinal motility	Reduced	Normal	Normal
Biliary function	Reduced	Normal	Normal
Microbial flora	Acquiring	Adult pattern	Adult pattern

From Michael D, Reed PG. Principles of drug therapy. In: Berhman R, Kliegman R, Jenson H, editors. *Nelson textbook of pediatrics*. 17th ed. Philadelphia: Elsevier Science; 2004. p. 2428–32.

Patient evaluation

Past medical history and physical examination constitute the two most important tools in oral and maxillofacial surgeons' armamentarium for the perioperative evaluation of pediatric patients and subsequent treatment. Details on history taking and pediatric physical examination are beyond the scope of this article and the reader is referred to other sources for their study.

During an interview with parents or legal guardians of children, careful review of the signs and symptoms of the current problem should be addressed. The history should include information regarding maternal habits during gestation, such as drinking or smoking. Maternal perinatal history and vaccinations should be questioned, especially when evaluating neonates and infant patients. Gestational age at birth, birth height, weight, and Apgar scores should be obtained from parents or patients' pediatrician.

Family medical history can be as important as the history of the present illness in pediatric patients. It can reveal medical details that can make physicians suspicious for particular medical problems. Parents can report specific medical problems or provide significant symptoms affecting any of the family members. Anesthetic complications, allergic reactions to specific medications, bleeding problems, and genetic antecedents should be considered and investigated further to rule in or out conditions, such as malignant hypertermia and blood dyscracias.

Vital signs should be recorded on the first appointment and before any surgical procedure. Vital signs ranges by age are demonstrated in Table 2. Weight and height should be recorded routinely and patients' values extrapolated to growth charts corresponding to the patients' sex and age group. Growth charts can be obtained from the United States Centers for Disease Control and Prevention (Fig. 2) [16]. These measurements are helpful in calculating BMI and medication dosages. At the same time, developmental, growth, and nutritional abnormalities can be detected by the use of these charts. Childhood obesity recently has become a health care problem in the United States, its prevalence doubling in the past 20 years [17]. In 2003, the United States Centers for Disease Control and Prevention, in the Pediatric Nutrition Surveillance System, reported an overweight prevalence of 14.7% in children between 2 and 5 years of age. According to the American Academy of Pediatrics, children who have a BMI-for-age at or above 95% are considered overweight. Children who have a BMI-for-age between 85% and 95% are considered at risk for being overweight. Cultural and environmental causes, such as the consumption of high-caloric diets and sedentary lifestyle, account for some of the common causes of this problem. Ethnic groups, such as African Americans and Hispanics, are at higher risks for childhood being overweight compared with white children [18]. A dose-dependent relationship is found between the development of childhood obesity and maternal smoking [19]. Childhood obesity is related to significant comorbidities, such as higher prevalence of type 2 diabetes, increased blood pressure, abnormally high lipids and lipoproteins, and the development of SDB and obstructive sleep apnea [10,11] and should be evaluated and considered carefully when evaluating and treating children affected by this problem.

Routine laboratory tests usually are not required for healthy children. Specific tests should be ordered for children who have significant past medi-

Table 2
Normal range of vital signs

Age	Heart rate (beats/min)	Systolic blood pressure (mm Hg)	Diastolic blood pressure (mm Hg)	Respiratory rate (breaths/min)
Premature infant				
1 kg	120–140	36–58	18–38	40
2 kg	120–140	50–72	26–46	40
Term infant	120	65–80	30–50	40
0–12 mo[a]	100–120	105	65	40
1–6 y	100	105–110	70	30
6–12	80	110–125	70–80	20

[a] 90th percentile.

Data from Magnuson DK. Neonatal and pediatric physiology. In: Greenfield L, Mulholland MW, Oldha KT, et al, editors. *Surgery scientific principles and practice*. 3rd ed. Philadelphia: Lippincott Williams & Wilkins; 2001. p. 1901–31.

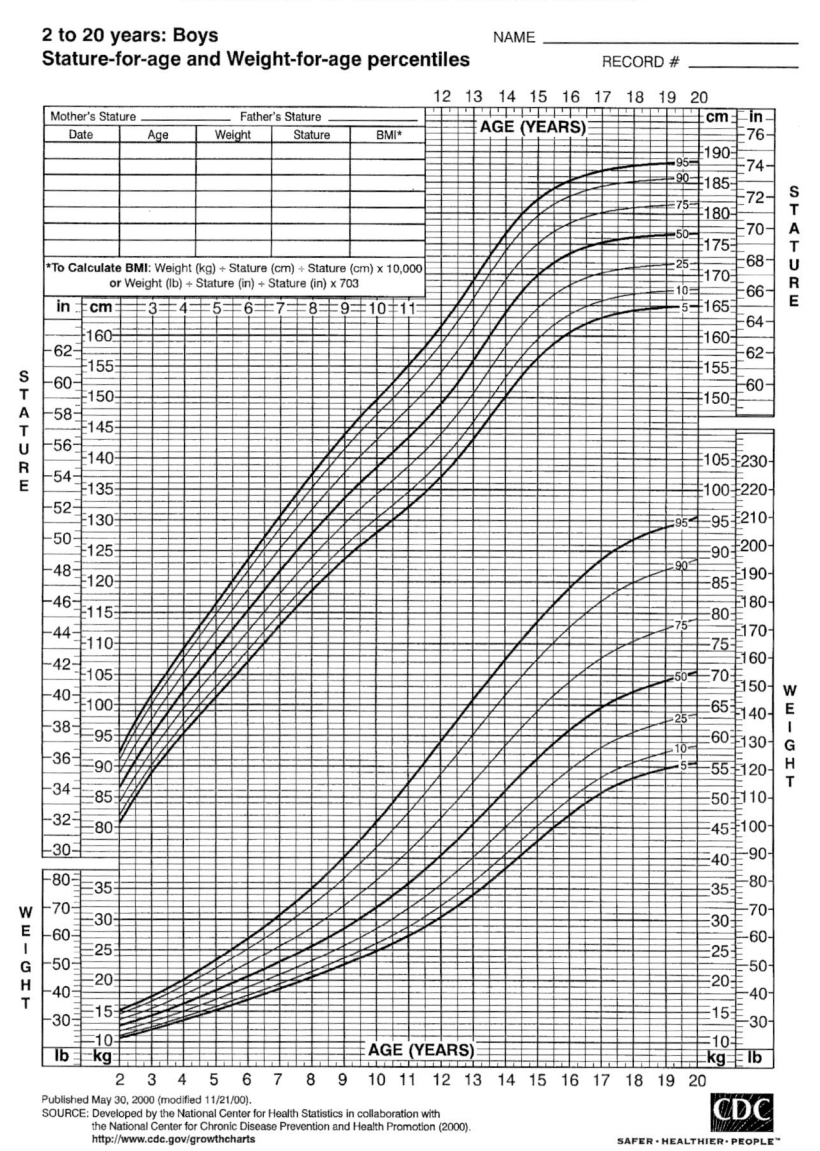

Fig. 2. Growth chart for boys between 2 and 20 years of age. (*From* The National Center of Health Statistics in collaboration with the Center for Chronic Disease Control and Prevention and Health Promotion; 2000. Available at: http://www.cdc.gov/growthcharts. Accessed April 8, 2005.)

cal or family medical history or positive findings on examination.

System-specific pediatric-related conditions

Respiratory

Respiratory infections

Children presenting with respiratory infections are at increased risk for anesthetic and postanesthetic complications [20,21]. This risk may continue for weeks after acute symptoms have abated. The intraoperative problems that occur usually are laryngospasm and bronchospasm, causing hypoxic events. Children normally are at higher risk for experiencing laryngospasm and bronchospasm. This incidence is increased with respiratory infections.

URIs, bacterial and viral, elicit an inflammatory response, which causes airway edema and increases airway secretions and decreased mucociliary clearance; the net effect decreases the airway lumen diameter. Airway reactivity also increases, leading to laryngospasm and bronchospasm. Airway hyperactivity can remain for up to 6 weeks after URI. It is recommended to delay elective procedures 4 to 6 weeks post URI.

Postoperatively, these children also may develop atelectasis. Postintubation strider occurs in 2% of all pediatric patients; this increases in patients who have URI. Tait and colleagues [22] show that children who have URI have a lower incidence of bronchospasm when managed with a laryngeal mask airway as opposed to being intubated with an endotracheal tube. These results suggest that sedations preformed without intubation may carry less risk.

Patients who have severe lower respiratory tract infections present a greater risk. Children having infections, such as pneumonia accompanied with fever, productive cough, or positive findings on radiograph, should have procedures delayed at least 6 weeks after convalescence. In contrast, mild coryzal symptoms, seen in patients who have allergic rhinitis, usually are not a contraindication to anesthesia [23].

Asthma

Asthma is a common childhood illness. The main types are atopic asthma, intrinsic asthma, and aspirin-induced asthma. Although each of these types of asthma has a different pathophysiology, they all represent a significant anesthesia risk. Studies show that 1.7% of patients who have asthma and have general anesthesia experience a severe respiratory outcome [24]. Because bronchospasm during a procedure or postoperatively may be disastrous, it is important to identify such patients with a thorough history and examination. In children, diagnosis is not always straightforward. Occasionally, cough may be the only symptom. Young children may vomit or have reduced appetite. Symptoms generally are worse at night; some patients may feel chest tightness in the morning. Signs on examination include expiratory wheezes and breathlessness.

Once identified, medical treatment should be maximized before a procedure requiring anesthesia. Achieving optimal control is paramount in avoiding perioperative complications. Before surgery, patients who have asthma should be asymptomatic by controlling medications and environmental factors. Medications should be continued and not held before the procedure. Prophylactic β_2-agonist agents may be given preoperatively to children who have mild disease.

Factors that increase risk in patients who have asthma include emergency department or hospitalization for acute attack within prior year, history of intubation, and prior treatment with systemic steroids. Patients who have more serious disease who are on steroids may need additional steroid support at the time of surgery. Steroids decrease edema and airway reactivity. Prednisone 1 mg/kg given at 24 hours and 12 hours before surgery may be used in these cases. Elective surgery should be delayed for children who are wheezing actively.

Intraoperatively, patients should be kept well hydrated. The airway should be suctioned thoroughly before extubation. Nebulizer treatments for postoperative wheezing may be given via endotracheal tube or mask. Postoperative analgesic medication containing aspirin should be given with caution as 10% to 11% of asthmatic patients [24] may be aspirin intolerant.

Cystic fibrosis

Cystic fibrosis is a fatal autosomal recessive disease, resulting from an inborn error of metabolism, causing dysfunction of all exocrine glands, leading to thickened gland secretions. Although many systems are affected, 90% of the related morbidity is pulmonary. The lungs eventually become progressively hyperinflated and mucus secretions become thick. This predisposes to infection and, ultimately, bronchiectasis. Pneumothorax and pulmonary hemorrhage are common complications. In addition to the increased anesthetic risk resulting from the pulmonary problems, perioperative management is complicated further by malabsorption secondary to pancreatic insufficiency, which leads to nutritional problems and electrolyte imbalances.

In general, patients who have cystic fibrosis are not candidates for office anesthesia techniques. Careful preoperative evaluation is necessary to avoid complications. Preoperative pulmonary function testing may be a useful predictor for postoperative mechanical ventilation in these patients [25]. Preoperative management includes, eradicating acute infections and treating bronchospasm with bronchodilators and steroids. Patients who have pulmonary-related heart failure need to be optimized with digoxin, diuretics, and drugs that decrease pulmonary vascular resistance.

Cardiovascular system

The depressant effects of most anesthetic agents combined with the diminished ability of the pediatric cardiovascular system to compensate stressful situations makes preoperative evaluation extremely important for children.

Murmurs

Murmurs are common in the pediatric population. Murmurs can be either innocent or pathologic. Innocent murmurs arise from cardiovascular structures in the absence of anatomic abnormalities. More than 30% of children have an innocent murmur at one time in their lives [26]. Innocent murmurs are accentuated during high-output states, such as fever, infection, and anxiety.

The most common innocent murmur is heard along the left midsternal border as a short systolic ejection murmur. Innocent murmurs that originate from flow into the pulmonic artery are heard best at the second left parasternal space and usually are a high-pitched and blowing type of systolic murmur. Venus hums also are considered innocent murmurs resulting from turbulent flow in the jugular venous system. These murmurs usually are heard anterior aspect at the of the upper chest or lower neck regions. Patients having these types of murmurs, who are asymptomatic and have a normal exercise tolerance, typically do not have increased anesthetic risk.

Pathologic murmurs include those that are diastolic, pansystolic, grade III or higher, harsh, located at the left upper sternal border, and associated with an early or midsystolic click or an abnormal second heart sound. Physical findings, such as cyanosis, weak pulses, and abnormal cardiac size on radiograph, often are associated with pathologic murmurs. Children having these types of murmurs should be evaluated further, as they may be manifestations of a congenital heart defect or underlying cardiac disease. Previously undiagnosed murmurs in children also be should evaluated in the preoperative period. Besides a thorough physical examination and an ECG, an echocardiogram usually is essential in working up these murmurs.

Mitral valve prolapse

The incidence of mitral valve prolapse (MVP) is approximately 2% to 3% [27]. In the pediatric population, this condition usually occurs in older children and adolescents. It is the result of myxomatous degeneration of the valve leaflets and chordae tendineae, allowing redundant mitral valve leaflets to bulge into the annulus. It is considered idiopathic in more than half of the diagnosed cases.

MVP usually is asymptomatic. Some patients report nonexertional chest pain and, rarely, syncope. A midsystolic click with or without a late systolic murmur, best audible at the apex, usually is heard on cardiac examination. Echocardiogram examination is common to confirm the diagnosis. MVP is associated with Marfan syndrome, von Willebrand's disease, and polycystic kidney disease. It also may be seen in patients who have pectus excavatum and scoliosis on physical examination.

Rarely, children who have MVP may have arrhythmias, including supraventricular tachycardia and premature atrial contractions. Ventricular arrhythmias also may occur. Surgical management concerns mostly are for prevention of subacute bacterial endocarditis (SBE).

Preoperative antibiotic prophylaxis for subacute bacterial endocarditis

Children who have any form of valvular heart disease, intracardiac ventricular septal or atrial septal defects, or intravascular shunts are candidates for SBE prophylaxis when scheduled for a procedure that may cause a transient bacteremia. These procedures include dental or oral surgical, sinus, genitourinary, and gastrointestinal operations. Oral intubation is not an indication for SBE prophylaxis; however, nasal intubation is associated with a transient bacterima [28] and requires preoperative antibiotics.

As discussed previously, all children who have undergone surgery to correct a congenital heart defect must be premedicated before bacteremia-producing procedures with antibiotics for life. Children beyond 6 months from surgical repair of atrial or ventricular septal defects or patent ductus arteriosus do not need antibiotic prophylaxis. Additionally, children who have innocent heart murmurs do not require antibiotic premedication.

The American Heart Association recommends antibiotic prophylaxis regimens [11]. The indigenous flora in the field of surgery determines the choice of antibiotic. It is important that prophylactic antibiotics be used only during the perioperative period to reduce the likelihood of microbial resistance. Oral antibiotics may be given 1 hour before a procedure. Parenteral antibiotics usually are given at the time the intravenous (IV) line is started. Prophylactic antibiotics usually are not given after 6 to 8 hours after a procedure [29]. It may be necessary, however, to continue antibiotics in to the postoperative period to treat an established infection.

Neuromuscular disorders

Children who have neuromuscular diseases require special consideration when planning a surgical procedure. Anesthetics may add to pre-existing muscle weakness requiring postoperative ventilatory support. Additionally, diminished airway reflexes and delayed gastric emptying increase the chance of aspiration and postoperative pulmonary sequelae. A common group of neuromuscular disorders affecting children is the muscular dystrophies.

Muscular dystrophy is a group of skeletal muscle disorders. They are determined genetically and characterized by progressive muscle weakness. Gene mutations encoding the dystrophin-glycoprotein complex are believed to be the cause of muscular dystrophy [30,31]. These diseases are progressive and usually manifest symptoms anywhere between infancy and adulthood. Many of the dystrophies are present in infancy but may be undiagnosed until children develop further and the disease progresses. A thorough history, therefore, should be taken in all children, including questions concerning delayed walking and speech and other developmental issues.

Duchenne's muscular dystrophy is one of the more common genetic diseases. It affects 1 in every 3500 males as a result of an X-linked recessive mutation. The disease begins in early childhood. Patients usually do not live much past the second decade. Death usually is the result of respiratory or cardiac failure.

Duchenne's muscular dystrophy is characterized by severe proximal muscle weakness, progressive degeneration, and fat infiltration of muscle. This causes a gradual deterioration of motor function. Patients also manifest kyphoscoliosis and restricted pulmonary disease. These features combined with sensitivity to nondepolarizing muscle relaxants [32] put these patients at risk for postoperative respiratory compromise and possible need for ventilator support. Careful use of nondepolarizing muscle relaxants is advised to avoid excessive postoperative respiratory complications.

Rhabdomyolysis with hyperkalemia, during general anesthesia, is another concern in patients diagnosed with Duchenne's muscular dystrophy. Succinylcholine and some inhalation anesthetics can promote massive rhabdomyolysis. Halothane, isoflurane, and sevoflurane all are associated with this condition [33] and should be avoided in these patients. Anesthetics with less risk include opioids, propofol, benzodiazepines, neuroleptics, and nitrous oxide.

One of the most serious potential complications facing children who have muscular dystrophies and have general anesthesia is malignant hyperthermia. There is an increased incidence of malignant hyperthermia in this population [34–36].

Malignant hyperthermia may manifest early as increased expired carbon dioxide, tachycardia, and muscle rigidity. As the condition progresses, there is a dramatic increase in aerobic and anaerobic metabolism. This results in an intense production of heat and lactic acid, causing respiratory and metabolic acidosis. The high temperatures are associated with hyperkalemia, hypercalcemia, and increases sympathetic response. In the late stages, cerebral edema, disseminated intravascular coagulation, and cardiac and renal failure occur.

Anesthesia should be approached with caution in these patients. A history of delayed motor function, even in female patients, may indicate an undiagnosed neuromuscular disease. Children who have history and symptoms consistent with a neuromuscular disease should undergo genetic testing for malignant hyperthermia associated mutations.

In vitro halothane–caffeine contracture testing of a muscle biopsy specimen also may be able to identify patients at risk [37,38].

Treatment for malignant hyperthermia involves the use of dantrolene sodium. Dantrolene administration is appropriate in cases of true malignant hyperthermia and malignant hyperthermia associated with myopathies [39]. Both seem to share the common final pathway of calcium-induced muscle hypermetabolism, which can be reversed by dantrolene.

Psychologic considerations in pediatric perioperative management

Preoperative anxiety

Patients experience preoperative anxiety approximately 1 week before surgery [40]; this can be a stressful period. Feelings of uneasiness, tension, and nervousness can be difficult for many adult patients. This also can be an intense time for children. Anxiety can cause an increased induction time and an increase in the amount of medication needed for induction. Children may display preoperative anxiety in a variety of ways, ranging from subtle changes in behavior to exceedingly evident displays.

There are many factors that have a bearing on preoperative anxiety, including age, temperament of the child, previous medical experiences, and the level of parental anxiety [41]. Children between ages 1 and 5 have the highest risk for preoperative anxiety. Some children who have developmental delays may have higher risks for anxiety beyond these ages.

The level of parental anxiety is a contributing factor in children's level of apprehension [42]. The parental effect is not limited to just the preoperative experience. It also can heighten postoperative anxiety in children. A British study of 100 parents of children scheduled for surgery finds that 42% of these parents have significant anxiety [43]. Mothers are found more pathologically anxious than fathers in this study.

The type and quality of the preoperative preparation by surgeons and he anesthesiologists can have a significant effect on the level of preoperative anxiety experienced by children. Many institutions have programs to prepare children for surgical, anesthesia, and hospital experiences. These programs take many forms, including tours of the operating room area and hospital children's floors and videotaped instruction with teaching sessions of coping skills. Parents usually are included in these programs, which also can help diminish the parental effect of children's anxiety.

Although there is some debate over which type of program provides the most anxiety reduction in children, it generally is agreed that these prehospitalization preparation programs are of benefit to reduce preoperative anxiety [44,45].

Parental presence in the operating room

One method for reducing preoperative anxiety is having a parent present in the operating room for the anesthesia induction. The efficacy of this technique is controversial. The use of this method varies from institution to institution. Although frequently used in North America, parental presence in the operating room is more popular in the United Kingdom, where outcome assessments tout its effectiveness [43,46]. This technique seems to work best when there already is a low level of parental anxiety and children are less than 4 years old [47]. Kain and colleagues compare the technique of parental presence in the operating room with premedicating children with oral midazolam [46]. All patients and parents participated in a preoperative preparation program 1 week before the scheduled surgical procedure. Results show that premedicating with oral midazolam is more effective in reducing preoperative anxiety in child patients and in parents than the technique of parental presence during induction.

Medical-legal aspects of having a parent present during induction also should be considered. Hospitals and practitioners may be held responsible for parents who are injured secondary to syncope. If this technique is used, a protocol should be developed to manage parents who disrupt treatment or refuse to leave the operating room after induction. As with many techniques, thorough patient and parent preoperative assessment and proper patient selection is important when considering parent presence in the operating room.

Attention deficit disorders: attention deficit disorder and attention deficit hyperactivity disorder

Attention deficit disorders are conditions characterized by an attention span that is less than expected for a person's age; there often is also age-inappropriate hyperactivity and impulsive behavior. Because of increased awareness by educators and the public, more children are being diagnosed with attention deficit disorders. The disorder affects 3% to 5% of all school-aged children and is 3 to 10 times more common in men than women. Attention deficit disorders often may continue into adolescence and adulthood.

Children who have a hyperactivity component are diagnosed as having attention deficit hyperactivity disorder. Other children who are primarily inattentive and do not evidence significant hyperactivity are identified as having attention deficit disorder, inattentive type. There also is a combined subtype that has features of both.

Children affected by this disorder present several management concerns. A good baseline evaluation and documentation of patients' behaviors and level of function are helpful before planning a surgical procedure. Associated conditions, such as depression, should be identified during the preoperative assessment. Preoperative consultation with patients' mental health therapists may be important especially in children who might need increased postoperative support or modification in their treatment regimen. These consultations also may be useful particularly in aiding in the selection of preoperative anxiolytic medication and postoperative analgesics, as some sedative medications may not be effective or may produce an idiosyncratic reaction in children who have behavior disorders [48].

In addition to these behavioral management concerns, there are anesthetic matters that must be considered in children who have attention deficit disorders. These concern primarily the medication used to treat these disorders. Pharmacotherapy usually involves the use of stimulant medication, such as methylphenidate or similar, longer-acting compounds. These drugs tend to have excitatory properties. Side effects that may accompany these types of drugs include reduced appetite, headaches, sleep disturbances, anxiety, irritability, and depression. Patients taking these medications also may evidence facial tics. Other physical signs include possible tachycardia, increased blood pressure, and arrhythmias. Although children taking stimulant medications for attention deficit disorders generally tolerate anesthesia well [49], caution should be taken with coadministration of pressor agents and monoamine oxidase inhibitors.

Methylphenidate may decrease the metabolism of some anticoagulants, anticonvulsants, and tricyclic antidepressants. Dosage adjustments may be necessary when given concomitantly.

Fluid and electrolyte management

As discussed previously, many organ systems are not fully mature at birth or even during the first months of infancy. Among them is renal function, which is decreased compared with adults. Lower glomerular filtration and decreased capability to concentrate urine are the most important physiologic differences in infants up to age 1. In addition, patients scheduled for any surgical procedure under sedation or general anesthesia present with a degree of fluid deficit as a result of nothing-by-mouth restrictions. Box 1 shows the most important goals of fluid and electrolyte maintenance.

Fluid therapy should be oriented to replace water losses that are measurable and not measurable and to maintain the daily renal water requirements. The goal in terms of renal water requirements is to allow the complete excretion of a solute load at an osmolality of 250 mOsm/kg. Urine output accounts for 60% of the total measurable water losses. In neonates and infant patients, water diffusion through the skin accounts for the most significant source of insensible water loss because of immature stratum corneum on the epithelium. Under normal temperature and humidity conditions, the insensible water loss through the skin is 7 mL/kg/24 h [15]. Tables 3 and 4 illustrate methods of calculating the maintenance water rate and maintenance fluid volume. The most reliable measurement to assess appropriate hydration in pediatric patients is urine output. Under normal renal function, values of 2 mL/kg/h and 1 mL/kg/h for urine output are desirable for neonates and infants, and toddlers and school-age children, respectively.

Daily sodium and potassium requirements are 2 to 3 mEq/kg and 1 to 2 mEq/kg, respectively.

Isotonic IV solutions with osmolalities approximating 285 to 295 mOsm are the ideal choice for fluid replacement. IV infusion of hypotonic solutions induces red blood cell lysis by mobilization of water intracellulary. One-quarter or one-half percent normal saline and dextrose 5% can be administered IV as replacement solution. The addition of 10 to 20 mEq/L of potassium chloride provides the daily potassium requirements.

Preoperative fasting guidelines

The American Society of Anesthesiologists and its task force developed a series of recommendations for preoperative fasting and the use of pharmacologic agents to reduce the risk for pulmonary aspiration.

These guidelines are intended for healthy patients undergoing elective procedures. They may not apply or may need to be modified in patients who

Table 3
Maintenance water rate

0–10 kg: 4 mL/kg/h
10–20 kg: 40 mL/h + 2mL/kg/h × (weight−10 kg)
>20 kg: 60 mL/h + 1 mL/kg/h × (weight−20 kg)[a]

[a] The maximum fluid rate normally is 100 mL/h.
Data from Greenbaum LA. Pathophysiology of body fluids and fluid therapy: maintenance and replacement therapy. In: Berhman R, Kliegman R, Jenson H, editors. *Nelson textbook of pediatrics*. 17th ed. Philadelphia: Elsevier Science; 2004. p. 242–5.

Box 1. Goals of maintenance fluids

Prevent dehydration
Prevent electrolyte disorders
Prevent ketoacidosis
Prevent protein degradation

From Greenbaum LA. Pathophysiology of body fluids and fluid therapy: maintenance and replacement therapy. In: Berhman R, Kliegman R, Jenson H, editors. Nelson textbook of pediatrics. 17th edition. Philadelphia: Elsevier Science; 2004. p. 242–5.

Table 4
Body weight method for calculating maintenance fluid volume

Body weight	Fluid per day
0–10 kg	100 mL/kg
11–20 kg	1000 mL + 50 mL/kg for each kg >10 kg
>20 kg	1500 mL + 20 mL/kg for each kg >10 kg[a]

[a] The maximum total fluid per day normally is 2400 mL.
From Greenbaum LA. Pathophysiology of body fluids and fluid therapy: maintenance and replacement therapy. In: Berhman R, Kliegman R, Jenson H, editors. *Nelson textbook of pediatrics*. 17th ed. Philadelphia: Elsevier Science; 2004. p. 242–5.

have pathologic conditions that affect gastric emptying and also in those cases when a difficult airway is identified.

According to these recommendations, clear liquids may be consumed up to 2 hours before the scheduled surgical procedure. The volume of the liquids ingested is not as important as the type. Breast milk is allowed up to 4 hours preoperatively for neonates and infants.

Fasting for 6 hours is recommended for milk formula, nonhuman milk, and solids. Fried and fatty foods may decrease gastric emptying. The amount ingested should be considered when establishing the appropriate fasting period for these types of foods.

Pediatric drug dosages

Several equations are formulated to calculate the medication dosages for children. As discussed previously, many physiologic factors found in different stages of growing children may affect the pharmacodynamics, pharmacokinetics, and, therefore, the dosage of any medication.

Two of the most widely used formulas, based on children's weight or age [50], are: Clark's rule: dose = (adult dose × weight in pounds) ÷ 150 lb; and Young's rule: dose = (adult dose × age) ÷ (age + 12).

The most accurate but, at the same time, most cumbersome method for calculating the medication dosage for pediatric patients is based on BSA. Multiple equations can be used to calculate the BSA based on patients' height in centimeters and weight in kilograms [51,52]. The BSA formula to calculate children's drug dosages is [50]: ([BSA of child] ÷ 1.73 m^2) × adult dose.

Legal considerations involved in pediatric care

Informed consent

The concept of informed consent implies a discussion that includes key elements, including treatment options, risks involved, possible complications, and an explanation of the risks associated with not undergoing recommended treatment. Typically, informed consent is a process that is between doctor and patient. At the conclusion of the process, patients usually are asked to attest by signature that they have had such a discussion with their doctor and understand the options and risks that were explained.

Informed consent for pediatric patients involves another party: parents. Other than in emergency situations, parents or legal guardians are given the responsibility for medical decision making for patients less than 18 years of age. Children may be more capable of participating in treatment decisions than previously believed [53]. Although children legally cannot give consent for themselves, depending on the age and development level of children, their assent to the planned treatment should be sought. This should be done by including children in discussions about treatment when appropriate. This is important when planning surgery for adolescent patients [54]. Including children in treatment discussions serves the preoperative patient preparation and helps reduce anxiety.

Although in general, parents or guardians are responsible for providing consent for minors, there are instances when patients who are less than 18 years old may consent for themselves. These instances vary from state to state and are based on local laws [55,56]. In general, minors are considered emancipated if they are legally married, are a parent of a child, or are financially independent of their parents. Minors who are enlisted in military service also may fall into this category. Some states allow unemancipated minors to consent to medical therapy in certain cases, such as contraception and termination of pregnancy [56].

Situations where the parents are divorced may complicate the informed consent process. This is of particular concern if the parents do not agree on the proposed treatment. In some circumstances, there may be limitations on noncustodial parents concerning decision making and visitation. It is helpful to identify custodial parents when reregistering children as patients.

It is assumed that parents or guardians make decisions in the best interest of the patient. This may not be clear in situations where children are perceived at risk because of decisions made by parents based on religious beliefs. Again, state laws differ in approach to these situations. Many hospitals have policies and particular consent documents based on local law to deal with such religious objections.

Emergency care

When patients who are unconscious or for some other reason are unable to give appropriate consent present in an emergency department, there is a concept of implied consent for emergency treatment. Practitioners are required to institute emergency treatment and procedures that are in the best interest of patients. This also is true for children who are seen on an emergency basis when parents or guardians are not present. Treating providers may initiate emergency procedures as deemed necessary. Concurrent with these measures, a reasonable attempt must be made to contact patients' parents or guardians. Many emergency departments and hospitals have policies that cover this situation. These may involve having another practitioner other than the treating provider agree that the treatment is appropriate and emergently necessary. Practitioners involved in rendering pediatric care should be aware of institutional and state regulations regarding emergency treatment.

Treatment of pediatric patients carries with it ethical and legal concerns for patients' rights, confidentiality, and parents' rights. Providers must evaluate and respect these concerns when planning treatment for children.

References

[1] Groopman J. The pediatric gap: why have most medications never been properly tested on kids? New Yorker January 10, 2005;32–7.
[2] Cote CJ, Notterman DA, Karl HW, et al. Adverse sedation events in pediatrics: a critical incident analysis of contributing factors. Pediatrics 2000;105(4 Pt 1): 805–14.
[3] Cote CJ, Karl HW, Notterman DA, et al. Adverse sedation events in pediatrics: analysis of medications used for sedation. Pediatrics 2000;106:633–44.
[4] Mallampati SR, Gatt SP, Gugino LD, et al. A clinical sign to predict difficult tracheal intubation: a prospective study. Can Anaesth Soc J 1985;32:429–34.
[5] Brodsky L, Moore L, Stanievich JF. A comparison of tonsillar size and oropharyngeal dimensions in children with obstructive adenotonsillar hypertrophy. Int J Pediatr Otorhinolaryngol 1987;13:149–56.
[6] Fishbaugh DF, Wilson S, Preisch JW, et al. Relationship of tonsil size on an airway blockage maneuver in children during sedation. Pediatr Dent 1997;19: 277–81.
[7] Greenfeld M, Tauman R, DeRowe A, et al. Obstructive sleep apnea syndrome due to adenotonsillar hypertrophy in infants. Int J Pediatr Otorhinolaryngol 2003; 67:1055–60.
[8] Uruma Y, Suzuki K, Hattori H, et al. Obstructive sleep apnea syndrome in children. Acta Otolaryngol Suppl 2003;550:6–10.
[9] Gorur K, Doven O, Unal M, et al. Preoperative and postoperative cardiac and clinical findings of patients with adenotonsillar hypertrophy. Int J Pediatr Otorhinolaryngol 2001;59:41–6.
[10] Wing YK, Hui SH, Pak WM, et al. A controlled study of sleep related disordered breathing in obese children. Arch Dis Child 2003;88:1043–7.
[11] Erler T, Paditz E. Obstructive sleep apnea syndrome in children: a state-of-the-art review. Treat Respir Med 2004;3:107–22.
[12] Gozal D, Burnside MM. Increased upper airway collapsibility in children with obstructive sleep apnea during wakefulness. Am J Respir Crit Care Med 2004; 169:163–7.
[13] Magnuson DK. Neonatal and pediatric physiology. In: Greenfield L, Mulholland MW, Oldha KT, et al, editors. Surgery scientific principles and practice. 3rd ed. Philadelphia: Lippincott Williams & Wilkins; 2001. p. 1901–31.
[14] Shank ES. Perioperative anesthetic and metabolic care of children and adolescents. In: Leonard B, Kaban MJT, editors. Pediatric oral and maxillofacial surgery. Philadelphia: Elsevier Science; 2004. p. 100–9.
[15] Coran AG. The pediatric surgical patient. In: Wilmore D, Cheung LY, Harken AH, et al, editors. Care of the surgical patient: perioperative management and techniques, vol. 2. New York: Scientific American; 1995. p. 1–28.
[16] Polhamus B, Dalenius K, Thompson D, et al. Pediatric Nutrition Surveillance 2003 Report. Atlanta: US Department of Health and Human Services, Centers for Disease Control and Prevention; 2004.
[17] Cash A, Blackett PR, Daniel M, et al. Childhood obesity: epidemiology, comorbid conditions, psychological ramifications, and clinical recommendations. J Okla State Med Assoc 2004;97:428–33 [quiz: 434–5].
[18] Crawford PB, Story M, Wang MC, et al. Ethnic issues in the epidemiology of childhood obesity. Pediatr Clin North Am 2001;48:855–78.
[19] von Kries R, Toschke AM, Koletzko B, et al. Maternal smoking during pregnancy and childhood obesity. Am J Epidemiol 2002;156:954–61.
[20] Martin LD. Anesthetic implications of an upper respiratory infection in children. Pediatr Clin North Am 1994;41:121–30.
[21] Parnis SJ, Barker DS, Van Der Walt JH. Clinical predictors of anaesthetic complications in children with respiratory tract infections. Paediatr Anaesth 2001;11: 29–40.
[22] Tait AR, Pandit UA, Voepel-Lewis T, et al. Use of the laryngeal mask airway in children with upper respiratory tract infections: a comparison with endotracheal intubation. Anesth Analg 1998;86:706–11.
[23] Cohen MM, Cameron CB. Should you cancel the operation when a child has an upper respiratory tract infection? Anesth Analg 1991;72:282–8.
[24] Forrest JB, Rehder K, Cahalan MK, et al. Multicenter study of general anesthesia. III. Predictors of severe perioperative adverse outcomes. Anesthesiology 1992; 76:3–15.
[25] Maxwell LG. Age-associated issues in preoperative evaluation, testing, and planning: pediatrics. Anesthesiol Clin North Am 2004;22:27–43.
[26] Pelech AN. The cardiac murmur. When to refer? Pediatr Clin North Am 1998;45:107–22.

[27] Freed LA, Levy D, Levine RA, et al. Prevalence and clinical outcome of mitral-valve prolapse. N Engl J Med 1999;341:1–7.

[28] Berry Jr FA, Blankenbaker WL, Ball CG. Comparison of bacteremia occurring with nasotracheal and orotracheal intubation. Anesth Analg 1973;52:873–6.

[29] Dajani AS, Taubert KA, Wilson W, et al. Prevention of bacterial endocarditis. Recommendations by the American Heart Association. JAMA 1997;277:1794–801.

[30] Durbeej M, Campbell KP. Muscular dystrophies involving the dystrophin-glycoprotein complex: an overview of current mouse models. Curr Opin Genet Dev 2002;12:349–61.

[31] Kudoh H, Ikeda H, Kakitani M, et al. A new model mouse for Duchenne muscular dystrophy produced by 2.4 Mb deletion of dystrophin gene using Cre-loxP recombination system. Biochem Biophys Res Commun 2005;328:507–16.

[32] Ririe DG, Shapiro F, Sethna NF. The response of patients with Duchenne's muscular dystrophy to neuromuscular blockade with vecuronium. Anesthesiology 1998;88:351–4.

[33] Obata R, Yasumi Y, Suzuki A, et al. Rhabdomyolysis in association with Duchenne's muscular dystrophy. Can J Anaesth 1999;46:564–6.

[34] Kelfer HM, Singer WD, Reynolds RN. Malignant hyperthermia in a child with Duchenne muscular dystrophy. Pediatrics 1983;71:118–9.

[35] Brownell AK, Paasuke RT, Elash A, et al. Malignant hyperthermia in Duchenne muscular dystrophy. Anesthesiology 1983;58:180–2.

[36] Heiman-Patterson TD, Natter HM, Rosenberg HR, et al. Malignant hyperthermia susceptibility in X-linked muscle dystrophies. Pediatr Neurol 1986;2:356–8.

[37] Heiman-Patterson TD, Rosenberg H, Fletcher JE, et al. Halothane-caffeine contracture testing in neuromuscular diseases. Muscle Nerve 1988;11:453–7.

[38] Larach MG. Standardization of the caffeine halothane muscle contracture test. North American Malignant Hyperthermia Group. Anesth Analg 1989;69:511–5.

[39] Loke J, MacLennan DH. Malignant hyperthermia and central core disease: disorders of Ca2 + release channels. Am J Med 1998;104:470–86.

[40] Johnston M. Anxiety in surgical patients. Psychol Med 1980;10:145–52.

[41] Kain ZN, Caldwell-Andrews A, Wang SM. Psychological preparation of the parent and pediatric surgical patient. Anesthesiol Clin North Am 2002;20:29–44.

[42] Bevan JC, Johnston C, Haig MJ, et al. Preoperative parental anxiety predicts behavioural and emotional responses to induction of anaesthesia in children. Can J Anaesth 1990;37:177–82.

[43] Shirley PJ, Thompson N, Kenward M, et al. Parental anxiety before elective surgery in children. A British perspective. Anaesthesia 1998;53:956–9.

[44] O'Byrne KK, Peterson L, Saldana L. Survey of pediatric hospitals' preparation programs: evidence of the impact of health psychology research. Health Psychol 1997;16:147–54.

[45] Kain ZN, Caramico LA, Mayes LC, et al. Preoperative preparation programs in children: a comparative examination. Anesth Analg 1998;87:1249–55.

[46] Kain ZN, Mayes LC, Wang SM, et al. Parental presence during induction of anesthesia versus sedative premedication: which intervention is more effective? Anesthesiology 1998;89:1147–56 [discussion: 9A–10A].

[47] Kain ZN, Mayes LC, Caramico LA, et al. Parental presence during induction of anesthesia. A randomized controlled trial. Anesthesiology 1996;84:1060–7.

[48] Marshall WR, Weaver BD, McCutcheon P. A study of the effectiveness of oral midazolam as a dental preoperative sedative and hypnotic. Spec Care Dentist 1999;19:259–66.

[49] Fischer SP, Healzer JM, Brook MW, et al. General anesthesia in a patient on long-term amphetamine therapy: is there cause for concern? Anesth Analg 2000; 91:758–9.

[50] Pradel ECHJ. Geriatrics, pediatrics and the gravid woman. Oral Maxillofacial Surg Clin North Am 2001; 13:119–30.

[51] Gehan EA, George SL. Estimation of human body surface area from height and weight. Cancer Chemother Rep 1970;54:225–35.

[52] Haycock GB, Schwartz GJ, Wisotsky DH. Geometric method for measuring body surface area: a heightweight formula validated in infants, children, and adults. J Pediatr 1978;93:62–6.

[53] Zawistowski CA, Frader JE. Ethical problems in pediatric critical care: consent. Crit Care Med 2003; 31(5 Suppl):S407–10.

[54] Kuther TL. Medical decision-making and minors: issues of consent and assent. Adolescence 2003;38: 343–58.

[55] Vukadinovich DM. Minors' rights to consent to treatment: navigating the complexity of State laws. J Health Law 2004;37:667–91.

[56] Diaz A, Neal WP, Nucci AT, et al. Legal and ethical issues facing adolescent health care professionals. Mt Sinai J Med 2004;71:181–5.

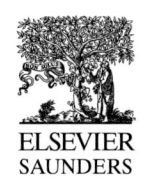

Postoperative Care of Oral and Maxillofacial Surgery Patients

Orrett E. Ogle, DDS

Department of Dentistry/Oral and Maxillofacial Surgery, Woodhull Medical and Mental Health Center, 760 Broadway, Brooklyn, NY 11206, USA

This article is aimed primarily at oral and maxillofacial surgery residents, recent graduates, and practitioners who do not manage hospitalized patients on a regular basis. Concepts of general care of surgical patients in the immediate postoperative period are related primarily to anesthesia issues, whereas later postoperative care is medical and surgical management. Because the perioperative care of patients who have specific medical problems is discussed in detail elsewhere in this issue, the postoperative management of patients who have medical problems, such as diabetes, cardiovascular disease, and so forth, are not addressed here.

The postoperative period begins when surgeons place the last suture and prepare to remove the surgical drapes. For most oral and maxillofacial surgery cases, the first postoperative concern is the removal of the throat pack if one was placed. Before a throat pack is removed, the mouth should be suctioned to remove debris and blood clots and the surgeon should keep the suction going until the throat pack has been removed fully. A good throat pack is one that, when removed, may be bloody or "dirty" at the oral end but generally clean on the tracheal end. The removal of the throat pack should be verified by the surgeon, circulating nurse, and anesthesiologist. The surface of the tongue should be wiped clean, as residual blood on the tongue may cause nausea and vomiting. After removal of the throat pack, some patients experience a sore throat, which usually disappears within a week. If the soreness is bothersome, over-the-counter lozenges containing a mild anesthetic can be used to provide temporary relief of the symptoms. Gargling several times a day with a mixture of 1 teaspoon of salt in 8 ounces of warm water can soothe the soreness temporarily and help flush out mucus if present. A cup of tea also may provide relief by warming the irritated membranes. The use of a humidifier or cool-mist vaporizer at night keeps the nasal and throat membranes moist and reduces the sore feeling.

At the termination of the procedure, the anesthesiologist must make a decision as to whether or not to extubate the patient and when the extubation should be done. Patients who have severe masticator space infections (Ludwig's angina) or acute facial trauma may have to be kept intubated and on a ventilator after their surgical procedure if a tracheotomy was not performed. Patients who have difficult airways that need special considerations include those who have had mandibular resections, neck dissections, uvulopalatoplasty, or maxillomandibular fixation. After temporomandibular joint arthroscopic procedures, surgeons should examine the oropharynx for swelling on the lateral aspects of the pharyngeal walls, because there may be partial or complete closure of the airway resulting from extracapsular extravasation of the fluid used to irrigate the joint during the procedure. Significant amounts of fluid can seep into the soft tissues medial to the temporomandibular joint and obstruct the airway [1]. Surgeons should examine the oropharynx and alert the

---

E-mail address: orrett.ogle@woodhullhc.nychhc.org

1042-3699/06/$ – see front matter © 2005 Elsevier Inc. All rights reserved.
doi:10.1016/j.coms.2005.09.005

anesthesiologist to any possible obstruction of the airway. Fortunately, fluids that seep extracapsular into the oropharynx dissipate within 60 to 90 minutes.

Most anesthesiologists do not like to do anesthetized extubations in oral surgical cases, but prefer awake extubation, in which patients are not extubated until they are judged ready to maintain and protect the airway, are responsive to verbal stimuli, and are able to lift their head. Common clinical criteria for extubation are

- Following verbal commands
- Having no active bleeding from the oral surgical site and no excessive or thick secretions in the oropharynx
- Sustaining head lift for 5 seconds or sustaining handgrip
- Having good breathing—respiratory rate less than 24/min; tidal volume greater than 5 mL/kg
- Maintaining oxygen saturation as measured by pulse oximetry (SpO_2) greater than 90%

The majority of nontraumatized patients who have oral or maxillofacial procedures are at low risk for postoperative respiratory complications, but they still require critical attention during the immediate postoperative period. Swelling of the soft tissues of the oropharynx and the floor of the mouth requires careful management of the airway. This swelling may not be manifested fully until approximately 12 hours postoperatively and may continue to increase for 48 hours after surgery. Luckily, the swelling is in the upper airway and not around the laryngeal inlet. Dexamethasone is used routinely to manage this problem in elective cases.

There are several aspects of postoperative care that merit specific discussion:

Ventilation and oxygenation

Because most oral and maxillofacial surgical procedures potentially can compromise the airway, special attention must be paid to maintaining a patent airway. It is the responsibility of oral and maxillofacial surgeons and anesthesiologists to assure that the airway is protected during and after surgery. Although patients may be strong enough to take deep breaths and may be awake, the ventilatory drive may not be adequate to maintain ventilation if drugs are interfering with the ventilatory center in the medulla. Anesthetic drugs shift the carbon dioxide response curve so that a higher carbon dioxide level is required to stimulate breathing. Inhaled anesthetics and barbiturates, benzodiazepines, opioids, and propofol all do this to varying degrees. Benzodiazepines and narcotics can be reversed, but barbiturates, the volatile anesthetics, and propofol lose their effects only through redistribution and metabolism. Assisted ventilation should be done until patients are able to maintain ventilation without an anesthetist telling them to breathe. Keeping the bed head elevated assists breathing and the management of oral secretions by patients. If it is necessary to reverse patients for respiratory depression with either naloxone (Narcan) or flumazenil (Romazicon), patients should be observed for at least 2 hours. The respiration again may become depressed because the half-life of the reversal agents are shorter than most opioids or benzodiazepines and their effectiveness diminishes after 60 minutes.

Inadequate respiratory drive after routine oral and maxillofacial surgical cases most often is drug related. Incomplete reversal of muscle relaxants is the most common cause in the hospital setting (oversedation is the most common cause in the office). When patients are not warmed during surgery and are cold, the reversal of muscle relaxants may not be complete, and cold patients that seem fully reversed can become reparalyzed as they warm up. When they are under anesthesia, there is vasodilation in the periphery, and as they emerge from inhalation anesthesia, the hypothalamus resumes its control; to conserve heat there is peripheral vasoconstriction. The peripheral vasoconstriction traps the muscle relaxant in the tissues, and as patients become warm and the vessels redilate, the muscle relaxant returns into the circulation and becomes active. Patients should be reversed adequately and kept warm.

Hypoxia is the major concern in the early postoperative period and its incidence is high. Xue and colleagues report that on room air, 30% of patients younger than 1 year old, 14% ages 3 to 14, and 8% of adults have hemoglobin saturation levels below 90% with many falling below 85% in the Post Anesthesia Care Unit (PACU) [2]. Anesthesia depresses respiration and produces ventilation-perfusion (V/Q) mismatch and pain and shivering that increase the demand for oxygen. Hypotension, hypovolemia, and severe anemia also reduce oxygenation of tissues further. V/Q mismatch mainly is the result of atelectasis and is a common cause of deoxygenation in the PACU [3]. After general anesthesia, there always is some degree of alveolar collapse resulting from a decrease in the functional residual capacity, which may take days or weeks to return to baseline [3]. Patients should be encouraged to breathe deeply and cough.

All patients require oxygen immediately postoperatively, but some high-risk patients may require supplemental oxygen for longer periods. Smokers, patients who have pre-existing pulmonary disease, elderly patients, patients who are morbidly obese, and individuals who have ischemic heart disease are at increased risk for hypoxemia [4] and should be given supplemental oxygen postoperatively until they are rewarmed, hemodynamically stable, fully awake, able to sit up, and pain free. Oxygenation should be monitored by measuring oxygen saturation (pulse oximetry). Oxygen at 40% by Venturi mask or 2 L/min by nasal cannula should be adequate for individuals who are not in severe danger of respiratory depression. In this high-risk population, swelling around the airway after major head and neck surgery may cause hypoxic episodes to develop during sleep for up to 72 hours after the immediate postoperative period.

Office-based anesthesia and conscious sedation are used widely in oral surgery practices, and postoperative considerations are different from procedures done in the hospital. Because the level of sedation usually is not deep, patients are aroused easily and can maintain their airway unassisted. High levels of oxygen given intraoperatively during oral and maxillofacial surgery office sedation contribute to the prevention of postoperative hypoxemia. Criteria for transfer from the dental chair to the recovery location are that individuals are capable of obeying verbal commands, are breathing satisfactorily, and have an oxygen saturation level greater than 95%. Because most of the agents used are short acting, patients return to their baseline of mental functioning quickly and generally can be discharged within 20 to 30 minutes after the procedure. For routine oral surgical procedures performed in an office setting under intravenous (IV) sedation, patients can be recovered with less monitoring and coverage. Complications that may have to be addressed postoperatively are emergence excitation, shivering, pain, episodes of nausea and vomiting, and, occasionally, oversedation.

Emergence excitation (dysphoria) is characterized by agitation and confusion. Although it usually is associated with emergence from ketamine or in patients who have received atropine or scopalamine (central anticholinergic syndrome), it also occurs often in patients who have not received any of these drugs. It seems to be more common in younger patients, with a higher incidence in females. In some cases, the agitation may be related to pain resulting from incomplete local anesthesia in lightly sedated patients.

Criteria for discharging patients after anesthesia or conscious sedation in the outpatient clinic at Woodhull Hospital are:

- Base line mental functioning is regained
- Stable vital signs are maintained
- Ability to walk with a stable gait unassisted
- Sufficient time has elapsed after the administration of reversal agents to ensure that patients do not become resedated after reversal effects have worn off

Postoperative pain management

Pain is unpleasant and unnecessary and its control must be a primary goal of postoperative care. It impairs oxygenation, delays healing, affects patients' attitude, and is a source of dissatisfaction with the surgical care. As there are no recognizable behavioral characteristics or clinical signs that can be used reliably to determine the actual degree of postoperative pain, it is best to believe patients' assessment of their own pain. The severity of pain towards the same surgical procedure varies among individuals and reactions to the same level of pain are expressed in different ways by different people. The best barometer of adequate analgesia, therefore, is patients' own perceptions. A scoring system should be used to assess the level of pain and to monitor the effectiveness of treatment. A reliable scale for acute pain [5] that is widely used is the visual analog scale (VAS)—the level of pain is determined by patients on a scale of 0 (no pain) to 10 (the worst imaginable pain). (Although the VAS is supposed to be a visual scale on which patients are asked to make a mark to represent the level of pain, they can be asked the level.) The Faces Pain Rating Scale (FPRS) [6] is a similar rating system more suitable for young children, as there is a certain amount of confusion in younger children (less than 7 years) when using the VAS [7]. In one study, it is the investigators' opinion that the FPRS is preferred by children and their parents and that this scale measures children's overall pain experience (ie, how "bad" they feel) more than the pain intensity. The VAS, in contrast, seems to measure only pain intensity [7]. There is no statistically significant difference between pain scores on the VAS or FPRS, however. The verbal rating scale is another scale that asks patients to rate pain intensity according to words, such as "none," "mild," "moderate," "severe," "extreme," and "worst ever" [8]. Most adult patients seem to prefer the verbal rating scale, because they are more comfortable using words than numbers to measure their pain [9].

Relief of pain reduces the sympathetic nervous system response and helps prevent hypertension, tachycardia, and other dysrhythmias. The use of IV opioids should start in the PACU soon after an anesthesiologist determines the level of arousal, orientation, and cardiovascular and pulmonary status. Premature use of parenteral analgesics or sedatives can worsen existing hypoventilation, airway obstruction, hypotension caused by central nervous system hypoxemia, incomplete recovery, and other conditions. It also is the responsibility of surgeons to assess the pain and provide patients with adequate and sufficient analgesics to permit continued pain control beyond the immediate postoperative period and for the succeeding 7 to 10 days. One study of postoperative pain reports that patients who have dental or orthopedic surgery complain of having higher incidents of pain compared to other surgical patients [10].

Pre-emptive analgesia

Pre-emptive analgesia (PA) is an evolving clinical concept that involves the introduction of an analgesic regimen before the onset of noxious stimuli, with the goal of preventing sensitization of the nervous system to subsequent stimuli that could amplify pain. Elective removal of third molars and implant surgery are two excellent settings for PA because the timing of noxious stimuli is known and the majority of patients are pain free before the procedure. When adequate doses of local anesthetic by infiltration, nerve block, or IV opiates are administered to appropriately selected patients before surgery, good pain control can be obtained for long periods after surgery. The most effective PA regimens are those that are capable of limiting sensitization of the nervous system throughout the entire perioperative period [11]. One of the most critical observations concerning central sensitization is the role played by the first phase of the pain response. Opiates administered before the first phase and reversed with the opiate antagonist, naloxone, before the expected onset of the second phase are shown capable of preventing the late stage of the pain response. Thus, preventing the initial neural cascade can lead to long-term benefits by eliminating the hypersensitivity produced by noxious stimuli [12].

The concept of PA is not accepted universally, however. Considerable controversy surrounds its use in clinical settings, because not all clinical trials of PA result in clearly defined advantages or of its effectiveness. Ko and colleagues [13] conclude from a double-blind, randomized control trial that PA is ineffective and does not reduce postoperative pain, the total number of analgesic doses per day, or the quantity of narcotic medication administered, nor does it shorten the length of hospital stay for patients who undergo appendectomy compared with healthy control subjects. They suggest that PA may be applicable only for patients who do not have preoperative pain. Aida and Shimoji substantiate the assumptions of Ko and colleagues. Aida and Shimoji [14] studied patients undergoing limb surgery and allocated the patients into PA or control groups. Pain was rated using the VAS. One group had presurgical pain (fracture surgery,and arthritis surgery), whereas the other had no presurgical pain (removal of orthopedic nails, bone plates, or a limb tumor). In the group of patients that did not have presurgical pain, they found that pain (monitored for 6to 48 hours after surgery) in the group that had PA was significantly lower ($P<0.005$) than those who did not have PA. Patients undergoing surgery who have PA used significantly less morphine ($P<0.005$) than those who did not have PA. Patients undergoing fracture or arthritis surgery who had PA, however, had no significant reduction in pain compared with those undergoing the same surgery who did not have PA. In fracture or arthritis surgery, there were no significant differences in morphine consumption between patients who had PA and those who did not have PA, and there were significant correlations between pre- and postsurgical VAS values in patients undergoing fracture and arthritis surgery who had PA. The greater the preopertive pain, the less success with PA. They conclude that central sensitization may be pre-established by presurgical pain and that presurgically imprinted central sensitization is preserved into the postoperative period and is not reversed by PA. The presence of presurgical pain, therefore, may be responsible for the controversy over the clinical validity of PA.

Another factor in the possible success of PA seems to be the duration of nerve block with local anaesthetics. A field block with bupivacaine induces PA after inguinal hernia repair and extraction of third molar teeth, whereas shorter-acting local anesthetics were less effective [15,16].

Successful strategies for using PA involve interventions at more than one site along the pain pathway. These strategies for pain related to oral surgical procedures include infiltration with local anesthetics, nerve block, IV narcotic, and anti-inflammatory drugs. For example, infiltrating the incision site with the long-acting local anesthetic, bupivacaine (Marcaine), after administering general anesthesia and before incision may offer benefits that last throughout the postoperative phase. Postoperatively, patients then could be given a nonsteroidal anti-inflammatory drug (NSAID) to control pain resulting from inflamation. Also, postoperative blocks with the longacting bupivacaine on completion of surgery also may contribute to long-term pain control in the postoperative phase. In an office environ where local anesthesia is the primary method of pain control, a NSAID could be given orally 30 to 60 minutes preoperatively and continued on a routine basis after surgery. A NSAID tablet given with a sip of water 2 hours preoperatively should not induce vomiting with IV sedation and should not prove problematic. It also is demonstrated that even if an NSAID is given up to 30 minutes after the procedure, before the effects of the local anesthetic wear off, it is effective in reducing pain [17].

Pain management in the majority of patients who have OMFS involves oral medications. Commonly used analgesics are described here.

Opioids

Weak opioids, such as codeine, dihydrocodeine, and, propoxyphene, have limited use on their own and are used best in combination with acetaminophen or aspirin. They are indicated for mild to moderate pain (eg, a pain score of 4 to 6) and cause nausea and constipation to the same extent as strong opioids without the analgesic benefit. Strong opioids, such as morphine, fentanyl, hydromorphone, oxycodone, and meperidine, are pure agonists that all have the side effects of nausea, vomiting, sedation, constipation, and respiratory depression. They are indicated for moderate to severe pain (pain score of 7 to 10). Morphine is the prototype of this group and is the drug of choice for postoperative pain in the hospital. It is administered in IV boluses of 0.05 to 0.1 mg/kg load then 0.8 to 10 mg/hour. The intramuscular (IM) dose is 7.5 mg for 75 to 140 pounds of body weight, or 10 mg for 141 to 220 pounds. Rarely, morphine can cause bronchospasm and, therefore, should not be given to patients who are wheezing actively. Although morphine can be used orally, its efficacy does not seem to be as good as when used parenteraly. Fentanyl can be given via a patch (every 3 days) for pain that is constant and stable.

Nonsteroidal anti-inflammatory drugs

NSAIDs are widely used analgesics shown effective for acute pain after oral surgery and are considered the drug of choice by many practicing oral surgeons. They are indicated for moderate pain and have good anti-inflammatory properties. All the NSAIDs work the same way and no particular one demonstrates superiority over others for pain relief, so two different NSAIDs should not be given at the same time. Not all patients react in a predictable fashion to the NSAIDs, however, so different ones may have to be tried.

A pain team, usually headed by an anesthesiologist with nursing specialists managing the floor operations, now exists in most United States hospitals. This team manages the acute postoperative pain of hospitalized patients and troubleshoots problems associated with acute pain management. Because the inpatient stay for the majority of oral surgical patients is short, surgeons should be involved so as to implement a satisfactory pain management regimen after discharge. Being involved alerts surgeons as to which patients may be difficult pain management subjects.

Unique postoperative pain management populations that require special consideration are children and the elderly. The major problem with treating pain in children is the difficulty of assessing their pain, particularly in those who cannot explain themselves. In very young children, observational measures are helpful. Assessing factors, such as whether or not the child is asleep, crying, relaxed, tense, or responding to their parents, can be used to create a cumulative pain score [18]. The absence of these signs, however, does not rule out the existence of pain or prove that the pain is controlled. Children over age 4 [19] are capable of reporting pain and, therefore, are able to use the FPRS.

The management of pain in children often needs direct attention from a caregiver. A strong effort must be made to observe children for signs of pain, as they may not be relied on for, or sometimes are incapable of, asking for analgesia when they are in pain; it may be better to establish a set schedule for analgesia [19]. The route of administration depends on the drug to be used, the severity of the pain, and the likely side effects. The oral route is preferred when possible but the rectal route may be used if the child is uncooperative or if vomiting is a problem. Acetaminophen is the mainstay of treating pain in children. It is effective for mild to moderate pain and can be given as an oral suspension in a dose of 10 to 15 mg/kg every 4 to 6 hours (to a maximum of 60 mg/kg in 24 hours). Slightly higher doses (20 mg/kg) are needed when used rectally as absorption is less reliable. Adverse reactions with acetaminophen are rare after appropriate dosing. The NSAID, ibuprofen, is available as an oral suspension or a flavored syrup and should be given in doses of 4 to 10 mg/kg, by mouth, every 6 to 8 hours to a maximum of 50 mg/kg/d. Aspirin never should be given to children under age 12 because of the association with Reye's syndrome.

Codeine can be given to babies or children who are outpatients by subcutaneous or IM routes and is effective for mild to moderate pain. Doses of codeine syrup for oral administration range from 0.5 to 1 mg/kg every 4 hours (not exceeding 60 mg per dose). Morphine given IV is the drug of choice for children who have severe pain and are inpatients. Normally, a loading dose is infused over 30 minutes followed by small incremental doses titrated against the child's pain and the presence of side effects. IV doses 0.07 mg/kg over 30 minutes as a loading dose and then 01 to 04 mg/kg hourly. Starting doses of analgesics for children are provided in the Agency for Health Care Policy and Research guidelines on acute pain management [20].

The elderly also present special problems in postoperative pain management. As a general rule, they report pain less frequently and often have multiple medical problems and many potential sources of pain. All this makes the assessment of postoperative pain difficult. The safe administration of analgesia to elderly surgical patients is complicated by chronic disease, polypharmacy, and nutritional alterations. The normal physiologic changes of aging alter the distribution, metabolism, and excretion of pain medication, thus affecting pain relief.

For most elderly inpatients, morphine is the opioid analgesic of choice [21]. Plasma clearance of morphine decreases as people age, so morphine remains in the body longer at higher concentrations. Propoxyphene and pentazocine should be avoided in elder patients, because propoxyphene has a toxic metabolite (norpropoxyphene) that relies on renal clearance for elimination, and pentazocine causes delirium and agitation in older adult patients. It is recommend that when administering opioids to the elderly, health care providers start with a 25% to 50% reduction of the recommended adult dose, increasing the dose by 25% on an individual basis while balancing analgesic need with undesirable effects. Dose increases are made based on individual reports of comfort and side effects, rather than on textbook recommendations of which milligram amount should be given [21].

Temperature

Patients lose heat during major surgery and may remain cold after the procedure unless active rewarming measures are taken. Hypothermia causes vasoconstriction and shivering, which feel uncomfortable, increase oxygen demand, and increase cardiac afterload. The muscle movement from shivering produces heat, utilizes glucose to produce carbon dioxide, and can increase oxygen consumption to the range of 135% to 486% of basal values [22]. Measures used to maintain body temperature in the operating room are an ambient room temperature and warm air blankets. Warm blankets or heated cotton sheets can be used to cover patients when they are transported to the PACU.

Temperature increases postoperatively should be categorized as (1) those occurring within 48 hours after surgery and (2) those occurring after 48 hours. Temperature increases in the first 48 hours postoperatively usually are caused by atelectasis. Measures to prevent this include deep breathing, early ambulation, intermittent positive pressure breathing, and adequate pain control. The fever should resolve with pulmonary toilet. A preoperative dental infection also may be the cause of early postoperative fever. Beyond 48 hours, some possible causes are wound infection, infection at sites of transcutaneous catheters, pneumonia, and urinary tract infection. All wounds should be examined, including IV sites, for signs of infection. Laboratory studies should include a complete blood count with differential, urinalysis, two sets of blood cultures taken from different sites during the febrile episode, and PA and lateral chest radiographs. The initial antibiotic treatment should be appropriate for the diagnosis. When diagnosis is uncertain, empiric therapy should be based on the most likely diagnosis.

Urine output

Oliguria is common during the immediate postoperative period. This may be the result of the response of the adrenal cortex to surgical stress and fluid and blood loss. There is an increase in antidiuretic hormone release (posterior pituitary) and aldosterone release (adrenal cortex) in the first 24 hours after surgery, which results in salt and water retention. Insufficient postoperative analgesia also can precipitate acute urinary retention because of the hormonal effects of the stress response. In addition, general anesthesia causes a decrease in renal blood flow and glomerular filtration rate. This postsurgical effect is temporary and should not last longer than 24 hours. Persistent oliguria (urine output less than 20 mL/h or 1 mL/kg/h in children) is related most frequently to hypovolemia. Urine output of less than 0.5 mL/kg/h for more than 3 hours may be indicative of acute renal failure (ARF).

Postoperative oliguria can be categorized as follows:

1. Prerenal azotemia: caused by decreased glomerular filtration rate secondary to hypovolemia or hypotension. This can occur secondary to blood loss, gastrointestinal fluid loss, excessive renal loss, and third spacing. The blood urea nitrogen:creatinine ratio is greater than 20. For optimum renal function, patients need to be hemodynamically stable with a near preoperative baseline blood pressure.
2. Acute tubular necrosis (ARF): often develops postoperatively when there is pre-existing renal disease, long periods of hypotension, use of nephrotoxic agents, septicemia, or hemolysis.
3. Other causes: (1) reflex spasm of voluntary sphincter because of pain or anxiety; (2) medications, such as anticholinergics and narcotics; (3) pre-existing partial bladder outlet obstruction, such as an enlarged prostate; and (4) mechanical obstruction, such as an occluded Foley catheter.

If patients cannot or have no desire to urinate after 2 to 3 hours postoperatively, consider that the oliguria is secondary to hypovolemia, as it is the most common cause of postoperative oliguria.

Treatment of postoperative oliguria is to first, relieve pain and, if possible, allow the individual to stand or sit to facilitate voiding. Then address the following:

1. Hypovolemia: treat hypovolemia, if identified, with boluses of normal saline (250-mL aliquots) until patients are maintaining urine output at 30 to 50 mL/h (adults) or 0.5 to 1 mL/kg/h (children). Diuretics worsen prerenal azotemia.
2. Mechanical obstruction: if there is mechanical obstruction, such as enlarged prostate, consider intermittent catheterization. If patients already have a Foley catheter, irrigate it to examine for obstruction.

NSAIDs can decrease urine output temporarily for a few hours after administration [23] and should not be given to patients who are oliguric, hypotensive, or hypovolemic. NSAIDs [23,24] and the selective cyclooxygenases cause prerenal ARF by blocking prostaglandin production, which also alters local glomerular arteriolar perfusion. Patients who have prexisting renal disease are at greater risk [23,25].

Nausea and vomiting

Postoperative nausea and vomiting (PONV) is a common, distressful, and debilitating occurrence that many patients describe as the most distressing part of their anesthetic experience. One study estimates it as affecting up to 35% of patients after day surgery [26] and that approxiamately 1% of patients undergoing ambulatory surgery are admitted overnight because of uncontrolled PONV [27]. In a hospital-based oral surgery practice Chye and colleagues report that the incidence of PONV after local anesthesia and IV sedation is 6% and 14% after general anesthesia [28]. Based on the numbers of people who have surgery annually, these reports suggest that millions of people experience PONV after general anesthesia or IV sedation.

Patients at higher risk for nausea and vomiting after surgery are children and young adults, women, those who are obese, individuals who are highly anxious, people prone to motion sickness, and those who have had nausea and vomiting with prior surgery. A higher incidence of PONV also is reported in women who are within the first 8 days of their menstrual cycle (highest at day 5) compared to those who were in the last portion of their cycle [29]. Smokers are less likely to suffer from PONV [30]. Patients undergoing surgery of the head and neck or intraoral procedures also may be at higher risk for nausea and vomiting. Ingestion of blood during and after intraoral or nasal surgery causes vomiting, which may raise venous and arterial blood pressure, which, in turn, may cause rebleeding from the surgical sites. Oral surgeons usually use a throat pack to prevent the ingestion of blood and avoid troublesome nausea.

Caution should be used with younger children, because they are prone to dehydration when they experience PONV from anesthesia or swallowed blood. Their oral intake may decrease significantly, because they are usually less cooperative about taking fluids than older children and their volume reserve is small.

Before giving antiemetics, consider if prior or existing medications may be causing the nausea, if it is secondary to swallowing blood, if an existing nasogastric tube is plugged, or if it truly is postanesthetic nausea.

Some useful drugs for PONV are prochlorperazine (Compazine), 5 to 10 mg IV every 6 h—may cause hypotension; metoclopramide (Reglan, Clopra, Maxolon), 5 to 10 mg (up to 30 mg) IV every 6 h; droperidol (Inapsine), 1.25 to 2.5 mg IV—may cause sedation; ondansetron (Zofran) 4 mg IV over 15 minutes. Prochlorperazine, metoclopramide, and droperidol may cause dystonia reactions, which may be counteracted by diphenhydramine, 25 to 50 mg IV/IM, or benztropine (Cogentin), 1 to 4 mg IV/IM.

Hemodynamic considerations

Routine, nontraumatic oral and maxillofacial patients do not present a great risk for being hemodynamically unstable. Basic situations are as follows.

The most common reason for postoperative hypertension is a preoperative history of hypertension. Other causes are pain, gastric or bladder distension, and fluid overload. The most common dysrhythmia is tachycardia. This is related mainly to pain but may be related to hypoxia or hypovolemia. Treatment is to identify and correct the underlying cause.

Wound care

Considerations of wound care are dependent of which part of the maxillofacial structure is involved and the type of wound (incisions, grafts, flaps, and so forth). Because of the variety of surgical procedures that are performed in the maxillofacial region, each with unique wound care requirements, only general principles are presented. The postoperative care of grafts or flaps is not discussed.

Postoperative considerations are

1. Minimization of bacterial colonization of the wound during the early healing period.
2. Prevention of trauma to the wound and immobilization of the wound edges. In general, facial incisions show no negative effect on healing from exposure. In fact, certain facial wounds must be exposed (eg, cleft lip or blepharoplasty incisions), because it is impractical to place a dressing [31]. Some patients however, are more comfortable if the wound is protected with a small bandage or adhesive skin closures to offer some protection from contact with bed linen.
3. The minimization of scarring by early removal of sutures as soon as the wound is strong enough to stay together—usually from 3 to 5 days for most facial incisions. Suture marks must be avoided meticulously. Collection of blood or serum around a suture as it passes out of the skin may cause a small stitch abscess, so it is important that the sutures are cleansed frequently and blood is not allowed to coagulate around them [31].

Sutures should be kept dry for the first 24 hours, after which time the face can be washed gently with a mild soap. The sutures should be patted dry right after washing with a clean towel. Skin wounds should be cleaned 3 to 4 times per day using a mild soap and water to wash the area around the wound, and a cotton-tipped swab dipped in a mixture of half water and half hydrogen peroxide may be used to clean the sutures. If secretions prevent adequate cleansing, then a light or water-soluble cream should be placed. When surgery involves a coronal approach, the scalp wound may be cleansed gently after 3 days. Hair should be kept dry until the day the stitches or staples are removed and then washed gently with baby shampoo.

Intraoral wounds present many challenges because of the need to ingest solids of diverse textures and various types of liquids at different temperatures. There also is the presence of multiple species of microorganisms that may cause opportunistic infections. The primary goal of intraoral wound care is to provide optimal conditions for the natural reparative processes of the wound to proceed. Patients should avoid disturbing the wound, particularly in the first 3 to 7 days. Mouth cleanliness is essential to good healing, as a clean wound heals better and faster. The mouth, therefore, should be cleansed thoroughly after each meal and individuals should rinse with warm salted water (one-half teaspoon of salt in an 8-ounce glass of warm water) 4 to 6 times daily until healing is complete. Patients should be encouraged to brush their teeth as best they can, particularly at bedtime. Dairy products should be avoided in the first 10 days. It also is best to avoid alcohol and tobacco for the first 2 weeks after surgery, as they make it easier for the wound to become infected and slow the healing process. The need for antibiotics for intraoral wounds should be a clinical one that is made on the basis of the type of surgery and its risk for becoming infected and the immune status of patients and the health of their organ systems.

In this issue of the O*ral and Maxillofacial Surgery Clinics of North America*, the majority of the articles discuss distinct aspects of perioperative care related to organ systems. The postoperative care of surgical patients, however, depends on the site of the surgery, the nature of the surgery, the type of anesthesia used, and comorbidities from diseases of major organ systems. Despite these variables, certain general principles are applicable and it is the objective of this article to present these principles. Care in the immediate postoperative phase and pain management are stressed, because these are considered the important aspects of postsurgical care.

References

[1] Handler BH, Levin LM. Postobstructive pulmonary edema as a sequela to temporomandibular joint arthroscopy—a case report. J Oral Maxillofac Surg 1993;51:315–7.

[2] Xue FS, Huang YG, Tong SY, et al. A comparative study of early postoperative hypoxemia in infants, children and adults undergoing elective plastic surgery. Anesth Analg 1996;83:709–15.

[3] Johnson SH, Plunkett MD, Gall SA, et al. The pulmonary system. In: Lyerly HK, Gaynor JW, editors. The handbook of surgical intensive care. 3rd ed. St. Louis: Mosby Year Book; 1992. p. 207–81.

[4] Xue FS, Li BW, Zhang GS, et al. The influence of surgical sites on early postoperative hypoxemia in adults undergoing elective surgery. Anesth Analg 1999;88:213–9.

[5] Bijur PE, Silver W, Gallagher EJ. Reliability of the visual analog scale for measurement of acute pain. Acad Emergenc Med 2001;8:1153–7.

[6] Wong D, Baker C. Pain in children: comparison of assessment scales. Pediatr Nurs 1988;1:9–17.

[7] Ostermueller KR. Comparative study of pain in hospitalized children and parental perception of that pain. FACES Research Abstract. Mosby Inc. 1988. Available at: http://www.mosbysdrugconsult.com/WOW/faces04.html. Accessed May 2005.

[8] Nierengarten MB. Commonly used pain scales valid measures of pain intensity. J Rheumatol 2003;30:509–11.

[9] Clark P, Lavielle P, Martinez H. Learning from pain scales: patient perspective. J Rheumatol 2003;30:1584–8.

[10] Chung F, Ritchie E, Su J. Postoperative pain in ambulatory surgery. Anesth Analg 1997;85:808–16.

[11] Gottschalk A, Smiyh DS. New concepts in acute pain therapy: preemptive analgesia. Am Fam Physician 2001;63:1979–86.

[12] Dickenson AH, Sullivan AF. Subcutaneous formalin-induced activity of dorsal horn neurones in the rat: differential response to an intrathecal opiate administered pre or post formalin. Pain 1987;30:349–60.

[13] Ko CY, Thompson Jr JE, Alcantara A, et al. Preemptive analgesia in patients undergoing appendectomy. Arch Surg 1997;132:874–7.

[14] Aida S, Shimoji K. Involvement of presurgical pain in preemptive analgesia for orthopedic limb surgery. Pain 1999;84:169–73.

[15] Atcheson R, Gill P, Kiani S, et al. Preemptive analgesia with bupivacaine following inguinal hernia repair. In: Devor M, Rowbotham MC, Wiesenfeld-Hallin Z, editors. Proceedings of the 9th World Congress on Pain, August 22–27, 1999, Vienna, Austria. Seattle: International Association for the Study of Pain; 1999. p. 580–4.

[16] Gordon SM, Dionne RA, Brahim J, et al. Blockade of peripheral neuronal barrage reduces postoperative pain. Pain 1997;70:209–15.

[17] Sisk AL, Grover BJ. A comparison of preoperative and postoperative naproxen sodium for suppression of postoperative pain. J Oral Maxillofac Surg 1990;48:674–8.

[18] McGrath PA. An assessment of children's pain: a review of behavioral, psychological and direct scaling techniques. Pain 1987;31:147–76.

[19] Varni JW, Walco GA, Katz ER. Assessment and management of chronic and recurrent pain in children with chronic diseases. Paediatrician 1989;16:56–63.

[20] Carr DB, Jacox AK, Chapman CR, et al. Acute pain management in infants, children, and adolescents: operative and medical procedures: quick reference guide for clinicians. Rockville (MD): Agency for Health Care Policy and Research; 1992.

[21] Pasero C, Reed BA, McCaffery M. Pain in the elderly. In: McCaffery M, Pasero C, editors. Pain: clinical manual. 2nd ed. St. Louis: Mosby; 1999. p. 674–711.

[22] Bay J, Nunn JG, Prys-Roberts C. Factors influencing arterial PO2 during recovery from anaesthsia. Br J Anaesth 1968;40:398–407.

[23] Thadhani R, Pascual M, Bonventre JV. Medical progress: acute renal failure. N Engl J Med 1996;334:1448–52.

[24] Shankel SW, Johnson DC, Clark PS, et al. Acute renal failure and glomerulopathy caused by nonsteroidal anti-inflammatory drugs. Arch Intern Med 1992;152:986–90.

[25] Griffin MR, Yared A, Ray WA. Nonsteroidal anti-inflamatory drugs and acute renal failure in elderly persons. Am J Epidemiol 2000;151:488–96.

[26] Carroll NV, Miederhoff P, Cox FM, et al. Postoperative nausea and vomiting after discharge from outpatient surgery centers. Anesth Analg 1995;80:903–9.

[27] Tramèr MR. A rational approach to the control of postoperative nausea and vomiting: evidence from systematic reviews. Part I. Efficacy and harm of antiemetic interventions, and methodological issues. Acta Anaesthesiol Scand 2001;45:4–13.

[28] Chye EP, Young IG, Osborne GA, et al. Outcomes after same-day oral surgery: a review of 1180 cases at a major teaching hospital. J Oral Maxillofac Surg 1993;51:846.

[29] Beattie WS, Lindblad T, Buckley DN, et al. The

incidence of postoperative nausea and vomiting in women undergoing laparoscopy is influenced by the day of the menstrual cycle. Can J Anaesth 1991;38: 298–302.

[30] Sweeney BP. Why does smoking protect against post operative nausea and vomiting? Br J Anaesth 2002; 89:810–3.

[31] Peacock EE. Wound healing and care of the wound. In: Kinney JM, Egdahl RH, Zuidema GD, editors. Manual of preoperative and postoperative care—American College of Surgeons. Philadelphia: W.B. Saunders; 1971. p. 1–18.

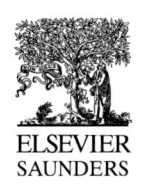

Psychologic Considerations in the Management of Oral Surgical Patients

Stanley Bodner, PhD

Adelphi University-University College, Department of Social Sciences, 1 South Avenue, Garden City, NY 11530, USA

Entering the often-sterile milieu that characterizes most surgical and presurgical environments sets into motion, for most patients, emotional or psychologic reactions. At times, these inner stirrings may manifest in the form of outward behaviors, such as expressions of anxiety or anger or verbalizations suggestive of depression. The essential psychologic issue is that undergoing any surgery—minor, major, elective, or urgent—is far from an emotionally neutral event for typical oral surgical patients.

Western society, in the twenty-first century, has grown more psychologically minded and sophisticated. If a more holistic approach is adopted regarding the treatment of oral surgical patients, it is anticipated that some tangible and intangible benefits will accrue. Specifically, practitioners can anticipate that with due attention to the psychologic needs of patients, there should be fewer preoperative, perioperative, or postoperative patient concerns and, perhaps, a corresponding decreased need for pain medication. In addition, patients can be expected to take greater responsibility for their own recovery, such as a commitment to greater compliance with postoperative care. Unfortunately, most oral surgeons devote their focus to their techniques and skills, giving scant attention to the biopsychologic factors apropos to a patient's perspective. If a purely mechanistic view of surgery is adopted, patients are more subjects than persons and, consequently, "the patient is seen as a passive recipient of a surgical intervention with little influence over the recovery process. Nothing could be further from the truth. Through psychological preparation for surgery, patients can be empowered to significantly impact their healing and recovery" [1].

Mechanic [2], an advocate of the biopsychologic perspective, suggests that patients' reactions to treatment, including impending or proposed surgery, at times, have little correlation with their actual physical disorder or disease process. Although biologic causes may stimulate nociceptive awareness, psychologic processes may affect the perception and interpretation of physical symptoms. Moreover, social variables, such as family and other support systems (or lack thereof), may moderate patients' actions or, for that matter, which interventions they allow to treat the origin of the pain.

The impact of emotions on oral surgical patients

In general, oral surgeons must be cognizant, to the extent possible, of the existing interplay between patients' emotions and their corresponding level of compliance, cooperation, surgical success, and recovery. The negative affect that patients experience can interfere with treatment compliance and due follow-up of treatment recommendations for maximum or speedy recovery. For example, patients who are unduly anxious may shun activities, exercises, surgical preliminaries, or postoperative recuperative actions, thus sabotaging maximum and efficient treatment

E-mail address: stanbodner@aol.com

effects. Depressed patients tend to feel helpless, lack a sense of self-efficacy, and exhibit a diminished drive to comply. Patients who vent anger at health practitioners or health care delivery systems tend to manifest a lack of motivation to follow suggestions or instructions proffered by health providers, as the latter are perceived as unempathetic, insincere, or condescending.

In the sections that follow, a research overview is presented designed to provide oral surgeons with a clinical "feel" for anxious, depressed, or angry patients, with the aim of sensitizing practitioners to important psychologic considerations so that surgical intervention can prove maximally efficacious, as far as circumstances allow.

Anxiety

Anxiety, or the experience of patient tension, may be transient, situation specific, or characterologic, that is, part of a defined or pervasive dimension of a patient's personality make-up. Transient, or situationally-based anxiety is conceptualized as a mental state of being. Anxiety that tends to be trans-situational is conceived of as a personality trait. Oral surgeons are challenged with patients who manifest anxious states and traits and must attempt to mitigate the sundry aspects of anxiety. The stress of an injury or disorder in the orofacial dimension can prove significant. Anticipation of, or actual oral surgery, with its frequent accompanying pain, engenders physical stress to the affected areas. Benson [3], who provides a body of literature and applications relating to the mind-body connection and the experience of stress, describes how body chemicals that stream from surgically impaired tissue sites can lead to additional decomposition of body tissue. This phenomenon can compromise individual immune systems and heighten the presence of stress hormones in the division that keeps the sympathetic nervous system activated. If patient stress is not addressed appropriately, surgical healing and recovery may be negatively affected or delayed.

In a seminal article on surgical stress, Kiecolt-Glaser and colleagues [4] assert that an inverse correlation exists between the degree of patient anxiety or distress experienced before surgery and the rate of postoperative recuperation. The greater the degree of presurgical anxiety, the slower, more delayed, and more complicated postoperative recovery is likely to be. Johnston [5] shows that highly anxious patients experience greater postsurgical pain. He points out further that, often, patients harbor particular concerns regarding surgery that are not shared with practitioners, including whether or not the surgery will be successful and how much postsurgical pain patients are expected to endure. Such concerns heighten surgical stress and can have an impact on presurgical, perioperative, and postoperative behavior.

Research in the area of psychoneurouimmunology shows that because surgery sets off a stress response in individuals, wound repair may be compromised [6–8]. Intense levels of presurgical stress are correlated with certain negative consequences, such as greater perceived postsurgical pain, longer hospital stays, higher frequencies of postsurgical complications, and greater levels of patient noncompliance [5,9]. Patients who have high levels of anxiety tend to require more anesthesia than their less anxious counterparts [5,10–12].

Various researchers (Kiecolt-Glaser and colleagues [13], Kiecolt-Glaser and Glaser [14], and Manyande and colleagues [15]) posit that efforts at altering patient perception, empowering patients with appropriate coping techniques, or shifting affect to a more hopeful stance has an impact on the immune or endocrine system in a way that stimulates recovery positively. Egbert and coworkers [16] provide a classic example of how psychologic intervention can serve to enhance surgical recovery. In their study, during the evening preceding surgery, anesthesiologists spent some time visiting their patients to clarify for them the type of pain sensations they should expect to experience postsurgically. In tandem with the anticipated pain sensations, the patients were taught relaxation techniques to help reduce the experience of pain sensation. The experimental group that was provided this presurgical treatment was discharged from the hospital, on average, significantly earlier and required approximately half the morphine levels of the control group. Additional studies emphasizing the positive effects of addressing the psychologic needs of surgical patients abound, providing ample evidence of stress reduction, reduced need for hospital care, greater patient compliance and follow-up, and reduced need for pain medication [11,17–21]. There are impressive studies that show that a significant relationship exists between patients' psychologic condition before surgery and their physical response during surgery [10,12,22,23].

In Johnston and Vogele's meta-analysis [18], correlations between various forms of interventions and the beneficial surgical outcomes are presented. Interventions, such as procedural orientation, sensory information, instruction in relaxation techniques, cognitive reframing or reconstructing regarding the surgical event, or hypnosis, in varying degrees, tend to modify the experience of pain, lessen the amount of pain medication required, reduce the average number of hospital days (if required), tend to show positive physiologic correlates and behavioral indicators of recovery, and bear positive feedback regarding surgical results. Contrada and coworkers [17], analyzing several studies focusing on presurgical intervention, find that approximately 67% to 75% of the experimental subjects, compared with controls, benefit from such intervention. Moreover, Contrada and coworkers find that when interventions, such as presentation of information relating to the various aspects of surgery, coping skills training, and the provision of emotional support, are combined, psychologic benefits to patients are maximized.

The benefits that derive from presurgical intervention, including brief patient-practitioner encounters, can prove impressive and invaluable. Devine [24], in a meta-analysis of 191 studies, finds that psychoeducational discussions and interventions undertaken with surgical patients for a median time of 30 minutes, yield shorter hospital stays in 79% of the studies and lead to the patient perception of less pain in a significant number of these studies. Not surprisingly, what generates anxiety in most instances is the patients' fear of pain. Oral surgical patients may have their nociception heightened through the subjective interpretation of pain, especially when patients experience undue presurgical anxiety. Vlaeyen and colleagues [25] find that with chronic low back pain, pain-related fear and avoidance behaviors designed to thwart pain actually intensify the perception of pain. In addition, Vlaeyen and Linton [26] and Vlaeyen and coworkers [27] advance the point that the pain experience, per se, stimulates negative cognitions and appraisals and may set into motion additional fears concerning the experience of sustained pain and the possibility of additional injury. It is of paramount importance for oral surgeons to be aware that often the fear of pain and the anticipatory anxiety concerning the pain experience are patient perceptions that do not necessarily match the actual nociception that should be experienced objectively. This, in turn, tends to have a negative impact on patient functioning, pain tolerance, and cooperation during surgery.

Because the experience of anxiety and pain perception are intertwined and because both factors can have a negative impact on degree of pain tolerance, level of patient compliance and cooperativeness, and speed and quality of surgical healing, it behooves oral surgeons to ascertain a sense of patients' pain fear before surgical intervention. Toward this end, there are several valid and useful psychologic instruments available to practitioners that can provide premorbid levels of anxiety. The Beck Anxiety Inventory [28] provides a good indication of patients' anxiety levels or whether or not patients may be suffering from a significant anxiety-related disorder (ie, whether or not patients' anxiety approaches clinical significance independent of concerns related to surgery). McCraken and Gross' Pain Anxiety Symptoms Scale [29] is a pain perception inventory that can serve as a useful tool in determining pain-related anxiety. Other suitable and valid instruments in the areas of pain perception, depression, somatization, and other psychically based disorders are discussed later.

To the extent that oral surgeons have some prior knowledge of patients' psychologic profiles, characteristics, or issues, they are in a better position to mitigate or plan for complications in the presurgical, perisurgical, and postsurgical phases of treatment. In some instances, when patients' psychologic issues prove to be profound in nature, such as in the case of body dysmorphic disorders, for example, a psychologic consultation is indicated with, perhaps, a consideration of postponing surgery.

The presence of depression

Sternbach [30,31] notes that the anxiety of acute pain is supplanted by the depression experienced with chronic pain. When patients present with comorbid dysthymia or depressive features in tandem with orofacial pain, it can be anticipated that patients' depressed affect intensifies the perceived pain, whether or not the pain is of an acute/transient nature, is benignly chronic, or is even more significant in degree. In actuality, pain and depression should be viewed as symbiotic or synergistic. Depressed affect exacerbates pain perception, and the experience of pain stimulates, intensifies, or exacerbates already existing depression or predispositions toward depressed affect. The pain perception-depression connection exists because depressed individuals have a proclivity to be withdrawn socially, to handle social interactions ineptly, to become avolitional and anhedonic, and to experience compromised mental processing. These consequences leave individuals feeling socially isolated and disconnected from others, with a negative self-perception and a negative "coloring," or interpretation, of external events. Given this mental state, perception of pain is magnified and compliance with presurgical instructions and the general interpretation of the surgical event may be affected negatively. Obviously, this can lead to surgical complications and poor surgical outcomes.

One valid and reliable instrument that can be administered easily to surgical patients is the Beck Depression Inventory [32]. This self-report instrument provides a rubric, with cut-off parameters, indicating patients' probable degree of depressed affect. With moderate to severe levels of depression, collaboration with a mental health practitioner may be essential for presurgical and postsurgical considerations. Given that epidemiologic studies show a high prevalence of depression in the general population, this issue cannot be eschewed in certain cases. One such study [33] determines that some level of depression affects as many as 10% of men and 20% of women during their respective lifetimes. In addition, as discussed previously, there is a greater presentation of depressive affect in patients who have chronic pain (which can include patients who present with oral or maxillofacial disorders) compared with patient populations who have no pain [34–37]. Patients who present with facial pain and temporomandibular joint disease also seem to show positive correlations with the comorbid presence of depression [38–41].

When working up patients' histories before proposed or impending surgery, patients should be appraised for evidence of depressive symptoms. If patients respond in the affirmative that they are experiencing sleep or appetite disturbances; have difficulty making decisions; seem anhedonic, anergic, or avolitional; engage in negative self-assignations; and report some degree of preoccupation with death, patients may be manifesting depressive symptoms. In more severe cases of depression, there are manifestations of either psychomotor retardation or agitation and expressions of delusionary thought. Such vegetative symptoms as psychomotor retardation or appetite disturbances tend to be observed in endogenous forms of depression. Instruments useful in pinpointing these symptoms include the Beck Depression Inventory or the Hamilton Rating Scale for Depression [42]. The latter is a useful tool for patients who have been diagnosed already with some degree of depression. The Postpartum Depression Screening Scale [43] is a self-report inventory that requires only 5 to 10 minutes of patient time to complete. Postpartum Depression Screening Scale items are sensitive to the presence of sleeping and eating disturbances, undue anxiety, emotional instability, insecurity, feelings of guilt and shame, and expressions of suicidal ideation.

Given the enormous time restraints that typical practitioners operate under, patients' completion of a depression screening instrument such as the Beck Depression Inventory, Hamilton Rating Scale for Depression, or the Postpartum Depression Screening Scale, may prove invaluable in identifying depressed patients or even serve to screen patients who harbor suicidal or homicidal ideation. Often, of course, a psychiatric consultation may be imperative upon discovery of signs of depression.

There are instances in which the early manifestations of a physical disorder present as depression. Unquestionably, the first step is to treat the underlying medical disorder. Although they are not the exclusive province of elderly patients, Salzman [44] points out that patients can present with depressive symptoms as a consequence of such physical disorders as: hypothyroidism or other endocrine imbalances; pernicious anemia; Parkinson's disease; intracranial tumors; various cancers; uremia or renal disease; electrolytic imbalances; or viral infections. Other conditions that often lead to depressive symptoms include Wilson's disease, myasthenia gravis, and emphysema. In some instances, depression may be secondary to a condition or disorder, and the depression may require concurrent treatment alongside the treatment of the physical disorder. Symptoms of depression also may be a consequent side effect of certain drugs that patients take for either acute treatment or maintenance, including medications such as reserpine, digitalis, L-dopa, corticosteroids, nonsteroidal anti-inflammatory drugs, and certain anticancer agents that might stimulate dysphoric mood [44].

Anger

Anger is an emotion often displayed by patients who are experiencing physical discomfort or prolonged distress as a consequence of chronic or recurrent pain [45]. Furthermore, with chronic pain patients it is not unusual to find that family members or caretakers harbor or express anger toward practitioners [46].

Physical or emotional factors that can contribute to the formation of internalized anger include: the presence of symptoms that patients experience as persistent and of long duration; the lack of understanding or knowledge regarding the cause of a given disorder; the experience of multiple treatment failures; the resentment bred toward employers, insurance companies, health care delivery systems, and their attending bureaucratic elements; and patients' awareness of the resentment felt toward patients by perceived unsympathetic family members. At times, patients engage in self-blame for being in their predicament. Any of these factors can singly, or in combination, lead to feelings of depression or anger, which can be either experienced internally or manifested as anger outbursts [47].

Kerns and colleagues [48] determine that patients' degree of unexpressed anger accounts significantly for patients' perceptions of pain intensity from a statistical standpoint. Fernandez and Turk [45] conjecture that anger magnifies perceived pain by stimulating patients' autonomic systems and serve to demotivate patients toward accepting practitioners' treatment plans and approaches toward recovery. In the case of chronic pain, where cure often is not attainable, patient anger compromises patients' levels of acceptance of available treatments or compromises their capacity to benefit from available care. Similarly, the suppression of expressed anger is correlated with poor treatment outcomes [49].

I suggest that practitioners elicit psychosocial information from patients or from key informants, when possible, as part of a new patient information work-up. If there is reason to suspect that patients harbor anger (regardless of source or target) during the presurgical process, and that the expressed anger or the indirect expressions of anger that are manifested (such as through the adoption of noncompliant behaviors or through negative attitudinal stances), it may prove difficult to achieve a good surgical outcome. Any effort on the part of health providers that can serve to assuage patients' negative emotions can serve only to make a surgical procedure, and patients' subsequent recovery, smoother, more successful, and, frequently, less painful.

Somatoform disorders or somatic complaints

There are patients who are predisposed to transforming emotional distress or tension into physical sensations or symptoms. Often, such patients seek out practitioners for medical attention [50]. In somatoform disorders (including conversion disorders, hypochondriasis, pain disorder, body dysmorphic disorder, and somatization disorder) [51], patients complain or present with physical symptoms that seem to have no organic basis. In such disorders, diagnostic tests cannot confirm a physical basis for the symptoms that patients manifest or claim to experience; yet, patients are not feigning, manipulating, imagining, or malingering with respect to the expressed symptoms.

Bodner [52] provides a useful overview of the various somatoform disorders, providing practitioners with a perspective as to how to address patients' needs before, during, and after surgery.

In conversion reaction [52], an extreme type of somatoform disorder, patient psychologic conflict is transformed, or converted, into physical symptoms or conditions, such as hysterical blindness or hysterical paralysis (such as "glove anesthesia"). Conversion reactions usually present subsequent to unrelenting stress or emotional trauma and competent mental health professionas can assist with differential diagnosis.

In somatization disorder [52], complaints generally are linked to a body system. Typical patients generally present, in seeming perpetual fashion, multiple and recurrent complaints, which can include various pain symptoms, dyspepsia or other gastrointestinal debilities, and such pseudoneurologic symptoms as selective anesthesia, diplopia or seizures. Karlsson and coworkers [53] estimate that approximately 20% of the patients who visit some form of primary care are, in fact, suffering from somatization disorder. Somatizing patients suffer significant negative self-bias when assessing their own health status [54], often experiencing some level of psychologic stress [55] (perhaps attempting thereby to obtain secondary gain, such as sympathetic treatment, from significant others), and exhibit exaggerated responses to normal sensory experiences [56].

Patients who have diagnosed temporomandibular disorder yield high scores on somatization ratings [57,58]. Reid and coworkers [59] maintain that in the case of masticatory muscle pain, patients have the tendency to experience heightened pain awareness. Schwartz and Gramling [60] argue that patients suffering orofacial pain benefit in the way of pain reduction when engaging in some form of cognitive behavioral psychologic treatment. Other studies [61,62] confirm that psychologic interventions, such as relaxation training, stress management, cognitive restructuring/reframing, and behavioral reconditioning, prove beneficial in the treatment of temporomandibular disorder.

A useful instrument that could assist in detecting the presence of a possible somatization disorder is the Symptom Assessment Questionnaire (SA-45) [53], which is a brief and valid, yet thorough, measure that identifies the presence of psychiatric symptomatology across nine psychiatric domains. The SA-45 can assist practitioners in making a differential diagnosis of anxiety-related disorders, depression, obsessive-compulsive disorders, exaggerated hostility, and so forth.

Certain surgical patients may present with hypochondriasis, wherein patients seem to be consumed with the fear that they will contract, or have contracted, a significant or malignant ailment, notwithstanding the absence of corroborative medical evidence [52]. In pain disorder [52], the pain is colored by an extreme subjective interpretation of pain, which can cause, or exacerbate, chronic pain. At times, patients are using the protective umbrella of a chronic pain condition to derive secondary gain from the added attention that others provide as they seek to comfort such patients. In body dysmorphic disorder [52], patients perceive some imagined defect or flaw in their appearance, especially in relation to a facial feature, such as the nasal or throat areas. This overabsorption with looks might lead to a series of unnecessary plastic surgeries or facial corrections.

Oral surgeons' appreciation of a somatoform disorder and the suspicion of the latter in a given patient's presentation (which can be supported or disconfirmed with an instrument such as the SA-45 or a psychologic consultation) can prove useful. Somatizing patients can present with remarkably realistic symptoms, and this accounts for why such patients may undergo twice the number of surgeries of patients in the general population [63]. In assisting surgeons in ascertaining if the source of orofacial pain is biogenic or psychogenic, it should be emphasized that, in somatoform disorders, the complaints of pain tend to be unusual or vague with respect to pathophysiology, or exaggerated—all with no, or little, organic basis [52].

Pretreatment considerations

Sword [64], in a well-known study, discusses the high level of stress experienced by oral surgeons and general dentists as they service their patient populations. Patient management and staff supervision are cited often as sources of stress for these professionals [65]. It is superfluous to state that oral surgeons are key with respect to ascertaining objective diagnoses, recommended treatment interventions, and expected prognoses. Nonetheless, patients' subjective interpretations and processing of presented information can determine whether or not they follow through with practitioners' treatment recommendations, including the role, function, and rationale for the proposed surgery. The surgeon must appraise patient's comprehension of the required or elective surgery and obtain a sense of patients capacities to cope with the stress of surgery.

More often than is appreciated is the frequent chasm between a surgeon's treatment plan and a patient's grasp of the value, necessity, and realistic results of an intervention or procedure. Ferguson [66] asserts that because patients often do not have sufficient understanding of the various aspects or the various facets of the impending surgery, the process of recuperation and healing is subject to complications. His reference to an American Medical Association report shows that as many as 58% of patient subjects believe that their doctors do not sufficiently explain important aspects of their condition and that only 31% of the subjects are willing to credit their doctors with providing ample time for preparation. Earlier studies conducted by Beckman and Frankel [67] point to the tendency of practitioners to interrupt patient queries within, on average, 18 seconds. Although this study is more than 20 years old, it probably would surprise no one if the findings were replicated in an updated study.

A related factor that serves to foster poor patient comprehension of impending surgery concerns the quality or efficiency of information transmission. Even if oral surgeons allow a reasonable period of time for patient-practitioner communication, patients frequently become mired in a jungle of jargon that serves to obfuscate and frighten. Sprinkling communications with "medicalese" can be expected to be related inversely to comprehension. In seeking to determine a psychologic motive, perhaps some practitioners unconsciously present surgical information in complex language either to impress patients with their knowledge or deter questioning, as patients may feel too embarrassed or intimidated to engage in much questioning. I have heard many patients slated for various types of surgery express, "I was too nervous to ask questions...I didn't really understand what he/she said, even though he/she explained a lot."

As a result of the lack of patient comprehension stemming from poor quality practitioner communication, temporomandibular joint, orthognathic, or other oral and maxillofacially procedures may be fraught with patient anxiety, which can serve only to impede optimal surgical outcomes [68]. In contrast, good surgeon-patient rapport leads to trust and patient cooperation, even if patients present with situational anxiety.

Expanded discussion

Johnston [5] asserts that better informed patients, presurgically, are patients who tend to fare well postsurgically; that is, being familiar with the upcoming procedure reduces complications during recovery.

Wallace [69] differentiates between procedural, sensory, and behavioral information. Procedural information essentially provides factual descriptions and explanations of what the surgery entails, the procedural sequence of the surgery, the rationale of the various aspects of the surgery, and the expected surgical process. Sensory information concerns the actual physical sensations patients should expect to experience during surgery and during postsurgical recovery. Behavioral information entails which specific activities or actions patients are expected to engage in, postsurgically, that help yield optimal surgical outcome during the recovery process and beyond.

The aim of having informed or educated patients is to foster an alliance with patients that, hopefully, serves to optimize the surgical outcome. Although this aim often is realized, there are some patients who seem to fare better with minimal information (patients should be allowed the choice). Miller [70] makes the distinction between persons who are either "monitors" or "blunters" in the face of a perceived aversive, noxious, or threatening event. Monitors seek to ferret out information concerning an anxiety-laden event, such as surgery, as this gives them a sense of empowerment or a perceived sense of control. Blunters, alternatively, choose to limit the amount of information the surgeons present regarding the upcoming surgery. Blunters may feel overwhelmed if given too much information about upcoming oral surgery and this, in turn, intensifies presurgical stress, which is correlated with poorer surgical outcomes (discussed previously). Unfortunately, blunters tend not to be stoical and choose to distort or deny, or even tune out, when surgeons attempt to impart information. Miller has devised a questionnaire which, in tandem with the direct query, "How much information, beyond the basics, would you like to hear about?" can serve to differentiate between monitors and blunters.

An issue of significance that tends to be glossed over by practitioners is the mistaken assumption that patients comprehend and retain information fully regarding the aspects or complexities of the oral surgery information explained to them [71,72]. Deardorf [1] asserts convincingly that only approximately 40% of patients read carefully the consent forms relating to procedures and their inherent risks, and only approximately 30% to 50% of patients are able to retain simple verbal explanations of the proposed or impending surgery. This figure improves only slightly when information is presented in written form. Most surgical consent forms or verbally presented information is too sophisticated and technical for the layperson. In addition, as most patients experience at least transient or situational anxiety, the processing of presented information regarding the surgery becomes diluted or distorted. Compromised comprehension of surgical procedures can lead to reduced presurgical and postsurgical compliance, which can, in turn, lead to less than optimal surgical results. Consequently, providers or designated assistants (ideally those who are attached to the surgical or procedural team) should make themselves available throughout the various phases of a surgical event, allowing for due attention to patient questions or concerns. Repetition of information should not stimulate practitioner exasperation; rather, it should be viewed as a necessary component of patient education and comprehension, which often is processed incrementally.

An important component of patient preparation is the necessity for providing an honest picture of what to expect or how patients are expected to feel postsurgically. In the absence of a complete or accurate postsurgical representation, patients are dependent on their own understanding or set of expectations with respect to the surgical outcome; at times, patient understanding may be rife with undue fear or unrealistic expectations. When necessary, practitioners should consult with significant others to ascertain how to present information or how much information to present to patients. In the area of postoperative or postprocedural pain sensation, patients should be given a realistic understanding of the discomfort they can expect in tandem with the palliative care that will be provided to help minimize or thwart pain or discomfort. As Deardorf [1] expresses cogently, when patients are not oriented with advance information regarding postsurgical pain and then they experience postsurgical pain, they becomes fearful that some aspect of the surgery went terribly awry and that the surgery was subpar or even calamitous.

Psychologic techniques useful for presurgical, perisurgical, and postsurgical patient preparation

Rugh and Solberg [73] point out that there is an impressive array of physiologic and psychologic interventions that have proven useful in the treatment of myofacial pain dysfunction, some of which are temporomandibular joint surgery, transcutaneous stimulation, pharmacologic intervention, occlusal adjustment, occlusal splints, clinical hypnosis, counseling, and biofeedback. Regardless of approach selected, Rugh and Solberg emphasize that successful practitioners are those who are able to demonstrate a psychologic "awareness" that is coupled with a willingness to listen and respond to patients' concerns.

Among the most effective psychologic approaches used in the brief treatment of presurgical anxiety or in coping with postsurgical pain management and recovery are the cognitive behavioral and relaxation strategies [74,75]. When necessary, these approaches are well suited for brief psychologic intervention.

During the past few decades, there has been a growing recognition that patients' cognitions are an important component to consider during the presurgical and recovery processes. The key assumption of all cognitive theories, pertaining to the understanding of anxiety, panic, depression, or pain, is that patient cognitions, perceptions, or interpretations serve as precursors in the formation of certain affective states. The objective reality of an event is not as crucial as patients' interpretation of the event. Oral surgical patients who believe in the capability of their surgeons and have an expectation of good recovery generally fare better than highly anxious, avoidant patients whose belief systems are characterized by pessimism or irrational expectations of surgeons or surgical events. In addition, the perception of positive self-efficacy, or patients' beliefs in their own capability in assisting their own recovery process, is an essential issue to consider. Turk and Rudy [76], in a comprehensive review of chronic pain studies, find that negative, maladaptive cognitions have an adverse impact on pain tolerance. Such negative cognitions include interpreting the healing environment as aversive or patients maintaining a low degree of self-efficacy.

In the cognitive behavioral approach, patients' cognitions are analyzed to ascertain how such thoughts serve to modify or intensify the experience of the nociceptive stimulus or the various aspects of the surgical process. Patient pain beliefs or appraisals relating to orofacial treatments or procedures often do not match actual nociceptive reality. Patients may interpret current conditions or disorders by equating physical sensations to prior experiences or by applying unrealistic expectations. Patients facing surgery generally experience some degree of tension and, consequently, may engage in negatively biased cognitions or what cognitive behaviorists' term, negative "self-talk." These are internally biased and often automatic cognitive interpretations that can serve to exacerbate presurgical and postsurgical stress. Maladaptive cognitions often are accepted, assumed, and automatic and may continue into perpetuity (trans-situational) unless questioned or challenged by patients at some point. In the absence of challenges or appropriate disputation, patients continue to accept these false cognitions or interpretations despite their potent illogic.

Deardorf [1] highlights some of the more frequent negative cognitions or biases in his article, suggesting the appropriate psychologic interventions to undertake when assisting surgery patients. These include castrophizing, filtering, black-and-white thinking, overgeneralizations, and shoulds.

When patients catastrophize, they imagine the worst possible scenarios or outcomes and proceed to act as though the outcomes are destined to occur. In filtering, patients attend selectively only to negative aspects or elements of situations and sacrifice or mitigate positive aspects or alternatives. In black-and-white thinking, a dichotomous or linear type of thought process is applied to objects, people, and activities (including surgery), with the former process perceived as either all good or all bad and an absence of a midrange or an in-between category. In overgeneralization, what is true of a single dimension of a situation is applied to all other dimensions or aspects of the situation, regardless of pertinence. In the shoulds, patients engage in irrational or inappropriate forms of self-talk. Should-type thinking leads to a listing of rigid and unrealistic rules about how individuals (including their bodies) and others "should" respond to a situation.

In a useful application of these cognitive errors or biases, Deardorf [1] presents examples of how surgical patients might engage in inappropriate cognitive distortion or self-talk. Thus, castrophizers might internally adopt the mental frame, "What if I never get better?" Filterers might internally maintain, "There is nothing that can help my situation." Black-and-white thinkers internally express, "The surgery either will restore me fully or be a failure." Overgeneralizers maintain, "Because I need this surgery, I will never be the same as I was...everything about me will be different." Finally, patients who have a should orientation might harbor the internal cognition, "I never should have allowed this to have happened!"

Catastrophizing is a common cognitive bias. Tripp and colleagues [77] find that individuals who have high levels of dental anxiety-catastrophyzing and pain-catastrophyzing tendencies experience higher subjective pain levels. Deardorf and Reeves [78] maintain that an important component of patient surgical preparation is assisting patients in identifying the type of cognitive bias or error they maintain internally and altering these negative cognitions through the technique of "stop-challenge-reframe." In this technique, the patients are taught how to isolate or recognize the negative cognitions harbored internally as they actually occur, then to challenge the inappropriate thoughts through logical disputation, and, finally, to replace the irrational or negative cognitions with healthier cognitions designed to help the patients cope more effectively. Through the use of a log or journal, patients can become adept in this technique, which, in turn, can serve to reduce anxiety or even depressed affect that present presurgically or postsurgically. When necessary, a brief intervention with a cognitive behavioral therapist may prove a useful adjunctive tool in the surgical process.

The use of relaxation techniques is applied extensively for the purpose of reducing presurgical anxiety or distress and for postoperative pain management. Among the various relaxation strategies that can be used preoperatively is progressive muscle relaxation combined with positive imagery, as these techniques have proved invaluable in the amelioration of stress and the postsurgical reduction of mild and moderate pain [79,80]. In an impressive study conducted by Thom and colleagues [81], patients who were dental phobic were provided with stress management and positive imagery techniques and were able to reduce their overall anxiety effectively compared with those who simply were administered benzodiazepine. Simple, brief techniques, such as mandibular or maxillary relaxation procedures, have proved useful in lessening subjectively perceived pain and reducing the need for an analgesic [74,75]. Turk and coworkers [82] find that patients who have temporomandibular disorder who are offered cognitive therapy in tandem with electromyogram frontalis biofeedback maximize treatment. In my experience, progressive relaxation procedures coupled with positive imagery instructions, but without biofeedback, show comparable outcomes. Clinical hypnosis and music-assisted relaxation also have proved efficacious in reducing presurgical stress [83,84]. Enlisting a psychologist for brief interventions can enhance patient compliance.

Factors that serve to complicate the surgical event

Malingering and secondary gain

Malingering tendencies on the part of patients have been given greater attention in recent decades. Malingering involves a purposeful attempt to deceive or produce an impression of a physical or mental disorder when, in fact, none exists. In legal cases, including disability or workers' compensation cases, patients attempt to fashion the impression of physical or mental incapacity or incompetency. The motivation for malingering and deceptive actions is tied to patients' desires to reap a possible financial windfall that might accrue, for example, in a personal injury settlement [85]. Surgeons might suspect possible malingering when patients, currently engaged in litigation or in a disability case, report more intensive pain and symptoms and with greater frequency, perhaps, compared with other patients who have no such backdrop or motivation. Similarly, recovery may seem to require a longer interval than practitioners expect [86].

A phenomenon related to malingering occurs when patients derive secondary gain by retaining the "patient label." The derivation of secondary gain serves as a disincentive for recovery from either surgery or the general treatment of an orofacial disorder. When patients, unconsciously, maintain the sick role because they are relieved from either work or domestic responsibilities, avoid interpersonal involvement or conflict, or receive additional special attention or fawning from target figures, they might be inclined to perpetuate symptoms or show less than full recovery.

Rogers [87] developed a highly valid instrument that assists in the identification or detection of malingering and deception that should be viewed as a useful tool in practitioners' armamentarium when grappling with the malingering dilemma.

Addicted patients

Bradley [88] has determined that approximately 20% of all visits to primary care physicians somehow are linked to alcohol or other drug-related issues. When patients seek the services of any health care provider, professionals have the need and responsibility to ascertain if patients present a history or a profile suggestive of substance usage. Oral surgeons may be confronted with situations in which patients present with a disorder or condition that is accompanied by reported pain. Generally, the report of pain is genuine, albeit, at times, exaggerated. At times, however, patients may be addicted to a prescription medication or an illicit drug. Practitioners may be challenged with making a judgment as to whether or not patients are expressing genuine pain sensation or are engaging in a form of manipulation so as to obtain pain medication.

Oral surgeons may suspect drug abuse when patients manifest at least several of the following symptoms [89]:

- Sleep difficulties
- Seizures

- Malnutrition and a wasting appearance, often accompanied by a pallor complexion
- Abnormal liver function, as reflected in blood chemistries and urinalysis
- Altered mood and affect, including displays of irritability, dysphoria, or anxiety
- Complaints of chronic pain that seem exaggerated or diffuse in nature
- Poor hygiene and self-neglect
- General restlessness and agitation
- Dry mouth and other anticholinergic symptoms
- Presence of nausea and vomiting
- Anorexia
- Slurred expressive speech
- Motor imbalance, tremors, shuffling gait
- Cigarette burns on fingers or clothing
- Unexplained bruises on parts of the body

In addition, rhinnorhea lacrimation, yawning, and vague complaints of muscle ache, especially along the extremities, are symptoms suggestive of withdrawal, typically from opiates or opioids.

There are several easily administered and easily scored screening instruments that can be incorporated into a patient's history work-up. Because patients who might be abusing substances typically engage in self-deception or denial, practitioners should explore the possibility of actual substance use when there is a basis for such concern. If clinical impression or judgment based on the presentation of patient symptoms leads practitioners to suspect possible use or abuse, toxicologic screening should be undertaken. When patients seem to be addicted to some substances, detoxification should be considered a primary step before surgery, provided the surgery is not in the nature of an emergency. When emergency surgery is required, important considerations arise relating to anesthesia and presurgical medications. For example, patients addicted to opiates or opioids often can be managed through administering 20 mg of methadone intramuscularly. As Nash and Hyde [90] caution, it is a surgeon's concern in treating opiate-addicted or opioid-addicted patients that there be no presurgical withdrawal.

Tables 1 and 2 [91–94] offer lists of some of the available biochemical and paper-and-pencil screening instruments that provide measures of liver function and other biochemical markers suggestive of alcohol abuse.

If health practitioners wish to administer only a brief screening instrument, the CAGE Inventory or Alcohol Use Disorders Identification Test (AUDIT) may be used. If more time is provided for alcohol screening, the Self-Administered Alcoholism Screening Test (SAAST) generally is suggested. There are instances in which the SAAST is completed by a patient's spouse. The Adolescent Drinking Inventory (ADI) is useful in identifying alcohol-related problems in teenagers who also might present with comorbid psychologic problems. When any of the alcohol screening instruments is used in tandem with biochemical screening tests, practitioners are given

Table 1
Biochemical screening tests detecting possible alcohol abuse

Screening test	Comment
Gamma-glutamyl transpeptidase (GGT)	GGT is a hepatic enzyme. GGT is the most widely used and one of the most accurate biochemical markers indicative of alcohol usage.
Aspartate aminotransferase (AST) and alanine aminotransferase (ALT)	These are hepatic enzymes necessary for amino acid metabolism. AST and ALT levels are elevated in the blood stream in the event of chronic alcohol consumption. Upon cessation of alcohol usage, AST and ALT generally return to normal levels.
Mean corpuscular volume (MCV)	This is a marker indicating heavy alcohol consumption. Elevated MCV may be reflective of alcohol's effect on red blood cells, folic acid deficiency, or significant liver disease. MCV is less sensitive than the GGT marker.
Carbohydrate-deficient transferrin (CDT)	Tranferrin is a glycoprotein that transports iron to body tissues. The carbohydrate composition of transferrin tends to be lower in active drinking. CDT has comparable sensitivity to GCT. Combining CDT and GGT heightens sensitivity without reducing specificity.

From Allen JP, Litten EZ. Screening instruments and biochemical screening tests. In: Graham AW, Schultz TK, Wilford BB, editors. Principles of addiction medicine. Chevy Chase (MD): American Society of Addiction Medicine; 1998. p. 203–71; with permission.

Table 2
Alcohol screening instruments

Instrument	Comments
CAGE Inventory	This is a brief, 4-item, self-report inventory that explores a patient's sense of the need to Cut down alcohol consumption, the experience of being Annoyed by others' critical of drinking behavior, the tendency to feel Guilty regarding consumption, and the need for an Eye-opener as a "starter" for the day.
Self-Administered Alcoholism Screening Test (SAAST)	Can be completed in approximately 10 minutes. The following aspects are assessed: loss of control; occupational/social disruption; negative physical symptoms; emotional disorder and pleas for help; other people's expressions of concern regarding the drinker; and familial conflicts with regard to the drinker's behavior.
Alcohol Use Disorders Indentification Test (AUDIT)	This screener was developed by the World Health Organization and assesses frequency of drinking, average consumption levels, and typical situations of abuse. The screener attempts to determine alcohol dependence or alcohol-related issues. There is a clinical examination section attached to the AUDIT inventory. Designed to achieve early detection of alcohol-related problems.
MacAndrew Scale	The MacAndrew Scale is a derivative of the Minnesota Multiphasic Personality Inventory (MMPI), which is one of the foremost and most valid of the personality assessment inventories. The MacAndrew Scale consists of 49 items. Some research shows that the scale appears to diagnose type I alcoholics with some degree of success [91,92]. The Substance Abuse Proclivity scale for adolescents is an adolescent version of the MacAndrew [93].
Adolescent Drinking Inventory (ADI)	A 24-item screening inventory geared to adolescent responders. This instrument is designed to isolate alcohol problems in teens referred for emotional or behavioral issues.
Alcohol Dependence Scale (ADS)	Has the focalized aim of determining alcohol dependence through ascertaining if the addicting elements of alcohol have "taken hold" of an individual. Thus, tolerance tendencies, surreptitious drinking behavior, and symptoms of withdrawal are explored.

powerful tools that can help identify an alcohol-related problem in surgical patients.

References

[1] Deardorf WW. Psychological interventions for surgery patients. In: Vandecreek L, Jackson TL, editors. Innovations in clinical practice: a sourcebook. Sarasota (FL): Professional Resource Press; 2000. p. 323–4.

[2] Mechanic D. The concepts of illness behavior. J Cronic Dis 1962;15:189–94.

[3] Benson H. Timeless healing: the power and biology of belief. New York: Scribner; 1996.

[4] Kiecolt-Glaser JK, Page GG, Marucha PT, et al. Psychological influences on surgical recovery: perspectives from psychoneuroimmunology. Am Psychol 1998;53:1209–18.

[5] Johnston M. Impending surgery. In: Fisher S, Reason J, editors. Handbook of life, stress, cognition and health. New York: Wiley; 1988. p. 79–100.

[6] Kiecolt-Glaser JK, Marucha PT, Malarkey WB, et al. Slowing of wound healing by psychological stress. Lancet 1995;346:1194–6.

[7] Marucha PT, Kiecolt-Glaser JK, Faragehi M. Mucosal wound healing is impaired by examination stress. Psychosom Med 1998;60:363–5.

[8] Padgett DA, Marucha PT, Sheridan JF. Restraint stress slows cutaneous wound healing in mice. Brain Behav Immun 1998;12:64–73.

[9] Mathews A, Ridgeway V. Personality and surgical recovery. Br J Clin Psychol 1981;20:243–60.

[10] Abbott J, Abbott P. Psychological and cardiovascular pre-dictors of anesthesia induction, operative and postoperative complications in gynecological surgery. Br J Clin Psychol 1995;34:613–25.

[11] Gil KM. Coping effectively with invasive medical procedures: a descriptive model. Clin Psychol Rev 1984;4:339–62.

[12] Markland D, Hardy L. Anxiety, relaxation, and anesthesia for day case surgery. Br J Clin Psychol 1993;32:493–504.

[13] Kiecolt-Glaser JK, Glaser R, Willinger D, et al. Psychosocial enhancement of immunocom petence in a geriatric population. Health Psychol 1985;4:25–41.

[14] Kiecolt-Glaser JK, Glaser R. Psychoneuroimmunology: can psychological interventions modulate immunity? J Consult Clin Psychol 1992;60:569–75.

[15] Manyande A, Simon B, Gettins D, et al. Preoperative rehearsal of acting coping imagery influences subjective and hormonal responses to abdominal surgery. Psychosom Med 1995;57:177–82.

[16] Egbert LD, Battit GE, Welch CE, et al. Reduction of postoperative pain by encouragement and instruction of patients. N Engl J Med 1964;270:825–7.

[17] Contrada RJ, Leventhal EA, Anderson JR. Psychological preparation for surgery: marshalling individual and social resources to optimize self-regulation. In: Maes S, Leventhal H, Johnston M, editors. International review of health psychology. New York: Wiley; 1994. p. 219–66.

[18] Johnston M, Vogele C. Benefits of psychological preparation for surgery: a meta-analysis. Ann Behav Med 1993;15:245–56.
[19] Johnston M, Wallace L. Stress and medical procedures. Oxford (England): Oxford University Press; 1990.
[20] Munford E, Schlessinger HJ, Glass GV. The effect of psychological intervention on recovery from surgery and heart attacks: an analysis of the literature. Am J Public Health 1982;72:141–51.
[21] Suls J, Wan CK. Effects of sensory and procedural information on coping with stressful medical procedures and pain: a meta-analysis. J Consult Clin Psychol 1989;57:372–9.
[22] Greene PG, Zeichner A, Roberts NL, et al. Preparation for caeserean delivery: a multicomponent analysis of treatment outcome. J Consult Clin Psychol 1989;57:484–7.
[23] Scheier MF, Matthews KA, Owens JF, et al. Dispositional optimism and recovery from coronary artery bypass surgery: the beneficial effects of physical and psychological well-being. J Pers Soc Psychol 1989;57:1024–40.
[24] Devine EC. Effects of psychoeducational care for adult surgical patients: a meta-analysis of 191 studies. Patient Educ Couns 1992;19:129–42.
[25] Vlaeyen JWS, Kole-Snijders A, Rooteveel A, et al. Behavioral rehabilitation of chronic low back pain—comparison of an operant, and operative cognitive treatment and an operant respondent treatment. Br J Clin Psychol 1995;34:95–118.
[26] Vlaeyen JW, Linton SJ. Fear avoidance and its consequences in chronic musculoskeletal pain: a state of the art. Pain 2000;85:317–32.
[27] Vlaeyen JW, de Jong J, Sieben J, et al. Graded exposure *in vivo* for pain related fear. In: Turk DC, Gatchel RJ, editors. Psychological approach to pain management. New York: Gulford; 2002. p. 210–34.
[28] Beck AT. Beck Anxiety Inventory. San Antonio (TX): Harcourt Assessment; 1993.
[29] McCracken LM, Gross RT. The Pain Anxiety Symptoms Scale (PASS) and the assessment of emotional responses to pain. In: VandeCreek L, Knapp S, Jackson TL, editors. Innovations in clinical practice: a source book. Sarasota (FL): Professional Resources Press; 1995. p. 309–21.
[30] Sternbach RA. Psychological aspects of pain and the selection of patients. Clin Neurosurg 1974;21:323–33.
[31] Sternbach RA. Psychophysiology of pain. In: Lipowski ZJ, editor. Psychosomatic medicine. New York: Oxford University Press; 1997. p. 98–106.
[32] Beck AT, Steer RA, Brown GK. Beck Depression Inventory. El Paso (TX): Psychological Corporation Assessment Catalogue; 2004. p. 117.
[33] Kessler RC, McGonagle KA, Zhao S, et al. Lifetime and 12-month prevalence of DSM III-R psychiatric disorders in the United States. Results from the National Comorbidity Survey. Arch Gen Psychiatry 1994;51:8–19.
[34] Dworkin SF, VonKoff M, Le Resche L. Multiple pain and psychiatric disturbance: An epidemiologic investigation. Arch Gen Psychiatry 1990;47:239–44.
[35] Lautenbacher S, Spernal J, Schreiber W, et al. Relationship between clinical pain complaints and pain sensitivity in patients with depression and panic disorders. Psychosom Med 1999;61:822–7.
[36] Magni G. On the relationship between chronic pain and depression when there is no organic lesion. Pain 1987;31:1–21.
[37] VonKorff M, Dworkin SF, LeResche L, et al. An epidemiologic comparison of pain complaints. Pain 1988;32:173–83.
[38] McCreary CP, Clark GT, Merril RL, et al. Psychological distress and diagnostic subgroups of temporomandibular disorder patients. Pain 1991;44:29–34.
[39] Gallagher RM, Marbach JJ, Raphael KG, et al. Is major depression comorbid with temporomandibular pain and dysfunction syndrome? A pilot study. Clin J Pain 1991;7:219–25.
[40] Korzun A, Hinderstein B, Wong M, et al. Comorbidity of depression with chronic facial pain and temporomandibular disorders. Oral Surg Oral Med Oral Pathol Oral Radiol Endod 1996;82:496–500.
[41] Madland G, Feinmann C, Newman S. Factors associated with anxiety and depression in facial arthromyalgia. Pain 2000;84:225–32.
[42] Reynolds WM, Kobak KA. Hamilton Depression Inventory. Lutz (FL): Psychological Assessment Resources Catalogue; 2004. p. 107.
[43] Beck CT, Gable RK. Postpartum Depression Screening Scale. Los Angeles: Western Psychological Services Catalogue; 2003. p. 84.
[44] Salzman C. Depression and physical disease. In: Crook T, Cohen GD, editors. Physicians guide to diagnosis and treatment of depression in the elderly. New Canaan (CT): Keats Publishing; 1998. p. 201–10.
[45] Fernandez E, Turk DC. The scope and significance of anger in the experience of chronic pain. Pain 1995;61:161–75.
[46] Schwartz L, Slater M, Birchler G, et al. Depression in spouses of chronic pain patients: the role of pain and anger, and marital satisfaction. Pain 1991;44:61–7.
[47] Lipowski ZJ. Somatization: the concept and its clinical application. Am J Psychiatry 1988;145:1358–68.
[48] Kerns RD, Rosenberg R, Jacob MC. Anger expression and chronic pain. J Behav Med 1994;17:57–68.
[49] Burns JW, Johnson BJ, Devine J, et al. Anger management style and the prediction of treatment outcome among male and female chronic pain patients. Behav Res Ther 1998;36:1051–62.
[50] Okifuji A, Turk DC, Curran SL. Anger in chronic pain: investigation of anger targets and intensity. J Psychosom Res 1999;61:771–80.
[51] American Psychiatric Association. Diagnostic and statistical manual of mental disorders. 4th ed. Washington, DC: American Psychiatric Association; 1994.
[52] Bodner S. Psychologic aspects of chronic pain. In: Dym H, editor. Oral and maxillofacial surgery clinics of North America: diagnosis and management

of facial pain. Philadelphia: Elsevier/Saunders; 2000. p. 181–202.
[53] Karlsson H, Joukamaa M, Lahti I, et al. Frequent attender profiles—different clinical subgroups among frequent attender patients in primary care. J Psychosom Res 1997;42:157–66.
[54] Katon W, Lin E, Von Korff M, et al. Somatization: a spectrum of severity. Am J Psychiatry 1991;148: 34–40.
[55] Mechanic D. Health and illness behavior and patient practitioner relationship. Soc Sci Med 1992;34: 1345–50.
[56] Blackwell B, De Morgan NP. The primary care of patients who have bodily concerns. Arch Fam Med 1996; 5:457–63.
[57] Wilson L, Dworkin SF, Whitney C, et al. Somatization and pain dispersion in chronic temporomandibular disorder pain. Pain 1994;57:55–61.
[58] McGregor BR, Butt HL, Zerbes M, et al. Assessment of pain (distribution and onset), symptoms, SCL 90-R Inventory responses, and the association with infectious events in patients with chronic orofacial pain. J Orofac Pain 1996;10:339–50.
[59] Reid KI, Gracely RH, Dubner RA. The influence of time, facial side and location side on pain-pressure thresholds in myogenous temporomandibular disorders. J Orofac Pain 1994;8:258–65.
[60] Schwartz SM, Gramling SE. Cognitive factors associated with facial pain. J Craniomand Pract 1997;6: 261–6.
[61] Turk DC, Zaki HS, Rudy TE. Effects of intraoral appliance and biofeedback/stress management alone and in combination in treating pain and depression in TMD patients. J Prosthet Dent 1993;70:58–64.
[62] Dworkin SF, LeResche L. Tempromandibular disorder pain: epidemiologic data. APS Bull 1993;3:12–3.
[63] Zoccolillo M, Cloninger CR. Somatization disorder: psychologic symptoms, social desirability and diagnosis. Compr Psychiatry 1986;27:65–73.
[64] Sword RO. Stress and suicide among dentists. Dent Surv 1977;6:12–8.
[65] Goodwin WC, Stark DD, Green TG, et al. Identification of stress in practice by recent dental graduates. J Dent Educ 1981;45:220–1.
[66] Ferguson T. Working with your doctor. In: Goleman D, Gurin J, editors. Mind body medicine: how to use your mind for better health. Yonkers (NY): Consumer Reports Book; 1993. p. 429–50.
[67] Beckman HB, Frankel RM. The effect of physician behavior on the collection of data. Ann Intern Med 1984;101:692–6.
[68] Bell R, Kiyak HA, Joondeph DR, et al. Perceptions of facial profile and their influence on the decision to undergo orthognathic surgery. Am J Orthod 1985;88: 323–32.
[69] Wallace LM. Psychological preparation as a method of reducing the stress of surgery. J Human Stress 1984;10: 62–77.
[70] Miller SM. Monitoring and blunting: validation of a questionnaire to assess styles of information-seeking under threat. J Pers Soc Psychol 1987;52:345–53.
[71] Ley P. Studies of recall in medical settings. Human Learning 1982;1:223–33.
[72] Roter DI. Patient participation in the patient-provider interaction: the effects of patient questions asking on the quality of interactions, satisfaction and compliance. Health Educ Monogr 1977;5:281–315.
[73] Rugh JD, Solberg WK. Psychological implications in temporomandibular pain and dysfunction. Oral Sci Rev 1976;7:3–30.
[74] Flaherty GG, Fitzpatrick JJ. Relaxation technique to increase comfort level of postoperative patients: a preliminary study. Nurs Res 1978;27:352–5.
[75] Wells N. The effect of relaxation on postoperative muscle tension and pain. Nurs Res 1982;31:236–8.
[76] Turk DC, Rudy TE. Assessment of cognitive factors in chronic pain: a worthwhile enterprise? J Consult Clin Psychol 1986;54:760–8.
[77] Tripp DA, Neish NR, Sullivan MJL. What hurts during dental hygiene treatment. J Dent Hyg 1998;72:25–36.
[78] Deardorf WW, Reeves JL. Preparing for surgery: a mind body approach to enhance healing and recovery. Oakland (CA): New Harbinger Publications; 1997.
[79] Lawlis GF, Selby D, Hinnant D, et al. Reduction of post-operative pain parameters by presurgical relaxation instructions for spinal pain patients. Spine 1985; 10:649–51.
[80] Horan JJ, Laying FC, Pursell CH. Preliminary study effects of "in vivo" emotive imagery on dental discomfort. Percept Mot Skills 1976;42:105–6.
[81] Thom A, Sartory G, Johren P. Comparison between one session psychological treatment and benzodiazepine in dental phobia. J Consult Clin Psychol 2000;68: 378–87.
[82] Turk DC, Greco CM, Zaki HS, et al. Dysfunctional patients with temporomandibular disorders: evaluating the efficacy of a tailored treatment protocol. J Consult Clin Psychol 1996;64:139–46.
[83] Locsin RG. The effect of music on the pain of selected post-operative patients. J Adv Nurs 1981;6:19–25.
[84] Kiefer RC, Hospodarsky J. The use of hypnotic technique in anesthesia to decrease postoperative meperidine requirements. J Am Osteopath Assoc 1980;79:693–5.
[85] Resnick PJ. Malingering of post-traumatic stress disorders. In: Rogers R, editor. Clinical assessment of malingering and deception. New York: Gulford; 1988. p. 84–103.
[86] Fee CR, Rutherford WH. A study of the effect of legal settlement on post-concussion symptoms. Anchors Emerg Med 1988;3:12–7.
[87] Rogers R. The structured interview of reported symptoms. Odessa (FL): Psychological Assessment Resources; 1992.
[88] Bradley KA. The primary care practitioners role in the prevention and management of alcohol problems. Alcohol Health Res World 1994;18:97–104.
[89] US Department of Health and Human Services—Substance Abuse and Mental Health Services Admin-

istration Center for Substance Abuse Treatment. Quick guide for clinicians, based on tip 26: substance abuse among older adults. Washington, DC: Department of Health and Human Services; 2001. p. 26. DHHS publication no (SMA) 01–3585.
[90] Nash GW, Hyde GL. Surgical management of the addicted patient. In: Graham AW, Schultz TW, Wilford BB, editors. Principles of addiction medicine. Chevy Chase (MD): American Society of Addiction Medicine; 1998. p. 859–61.
[91] Von Knorring AL, Bohman M, Von Knorring L, et al. Platelet MAO activity as a biological marker in subgroups of alcoholism. Acta Psychiatr Scand 1985;72: 51–8.
[92] Cloninger CT. Neurogenetic adaptive mechanisms in alcoholism. Science 1987;236:410–6.
[93] Colligan RC, Offord KP. MacAndrew versus MacAndrew: the relative efficacy of the MAC and SAP scales for the MMPI in screening male adolescents for substance misuse. J Pers Assess 1990;55:708–16.
[94] Stein SJ. MHS-Multi Health System Annual Catalogue—Symptom Assessment Questionnaire (SA-45). Tonawanda (NY): MHS Publishing; 2005. p. 73.

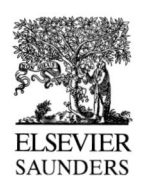

Fever Work-Up and Management in Postsurgical Oral and Maxillofacial Surgery Patients

Ryaz Ansari, BSc, DDS

Private Practice, 483 West Middle Turnpike, Suite 102, Manchester, CT 06040, USA

Humanity has but three great enemies: Fever, famine and war. Of these, by far the greatest, By far the most terrible, is fever.

Sir William Osler

This article focuses on the etiology, diagnosis, and management of fever in postoperative oral and maxillofacial surgery patients. A list of the causes of postoperative fever can be exhaustive. This article focuses on the more common presentations relevant to oral and maxillofacial surgeons. Some rare but important causes also are discussed. To be comprehensive in covering this topic, a definition of fever and an overview of its pathophysiology are included.

Definition of fever

Normal body temperature has a diurnal variation, with the lowest oral temperature at 6:00 AM and the maximum at 4:00 PM. Fever is defined as a temperature of greater than 37.2°C (99°F) in the early morning or greater than 37.7°C (100°F) in the late afternoon [1]. The operational definition of fever proposed by a consensus conference on sepsis and inflammation, however, is a body temperature greater than 38°C (100°F) [2]. For postoperative patients, an immediate work-up generally is recommended for any fever greater than 101.6°F after a single dose of acetaminophen on the first postoperative night or any fever greater than 101.6°F thereafter [3].

E-mail address: DocAnsari@hotmail.com

It should be noted that the terms, fever, hyperthermia, and hyperpyrexia, are not synonymous. Although all three conditions result in elevated body temperatures, fever results from the resetting of the hypothalamic center at a higher level in response to pyrogens (fever causing substances). Fever is a sign of inflammation (not infection); it is a response to the release of inflammatory cytokines (ie, tumor necrosis factor and interleukin [IL] 1β). In contrasting, in hyperthermia, the setting of the hypothalamic center remains unchanged, whereas body temperature increases uncontrollably, beyond the body's ability to compensate by losing heat. Examples of causes of hyperthermia are heat stroke, neuroleptic malignant syndrome, and malignant hyperthermia. The term, hyperpyrexia, is used for excessively high fevers greater than 41.5°C. This is seen in patients who have severe infections or, more commonly, in patients who have central nervous system hemorrhages. These distinctions are important not only in diagnosing the cause of fever but also in its management.

Chemical mediators of fever

Pyrogen is the term given to substances that cause fever. They may be exogenous or endogenous. Exogenous pyrogens are from outside the host, mostly of microbial origin, known as toxins. Endogenous pyrogens also are known as pyrogenic cytokines. Cytokines are small proteins that regulate immune, inflammatory, and hematopoietic processes. Some cytokines cause fever and, hence, are referred to as pyrogenic cytokines. These are IL-1, IL-6, and tumor necrosis factor. The production of these py-

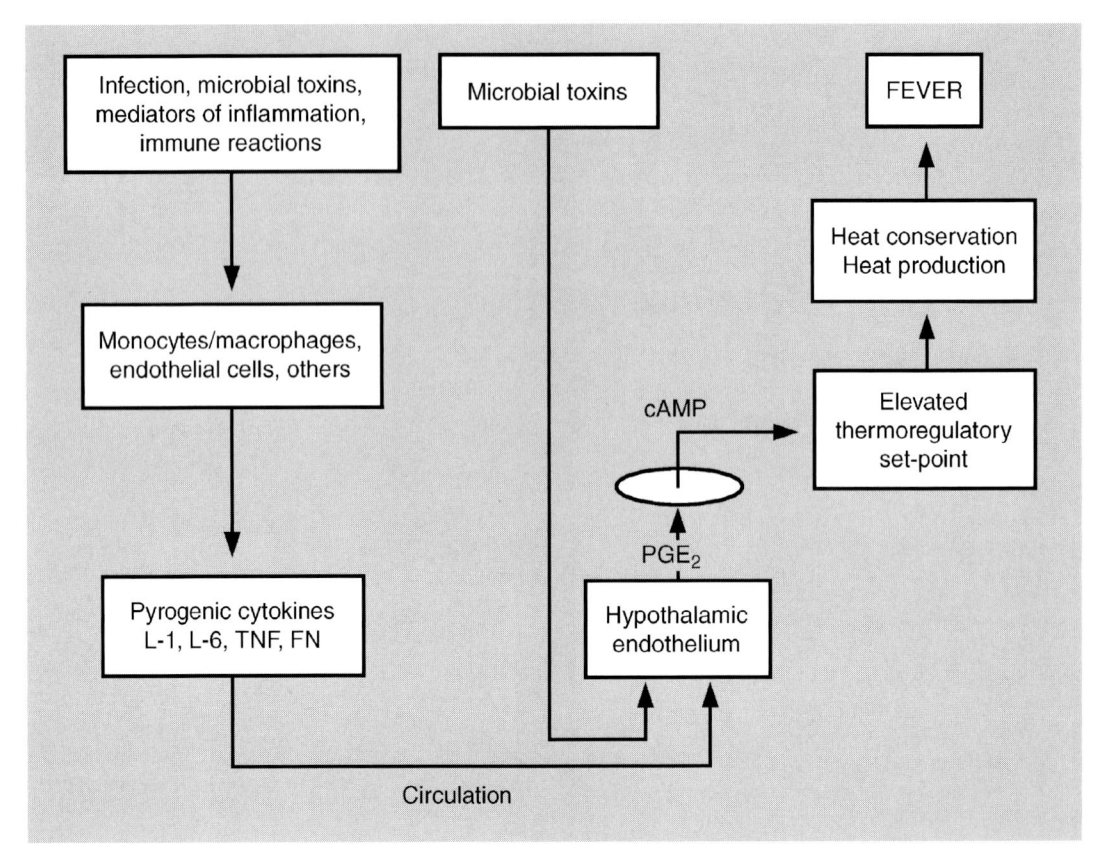

Fig. 1. From upper left, infections, microbial toxins, and other macrophage activators stimulate the production of pyrogenic cytokines. These, in turn, gain access to the circulation and interact with specific receptors (each cytokine has its own receptor) on the hypothalamic endothelium. In addition, microbial toxins can trigger receptors directly on the same endothelium in the hypothalamus and these receptors also are specific for each class of toxins. The response of the hypothalamic endothelium to either cytokines or toxins is the same, that is, the production of PGE$_2$. Cyclic adenosine monophosphate (cAMP) is released by PGE$_2$ and acts as a neurotransmitter. Elevated cAMP raises the set point and triggers peripheral heat conservation and production. (*From* Porat R, Charles D. Pathopysiology and treatment of fever in adults. In: Uptodate patient information, version 13.1; with permission.)

rogenic cytokines can be stimulated by infectious processes, trauma, or the presence of antigen-antibody complexes. The resulting cytokines then trigger the production of prostaglandin E2 (PGE$_2$) in the brain, which in turn acts on the hypothalamus to raise the setting in the hypothalamic centers to febrile levels (Fig. 1) [4]. The body responds with reflexive heat retention measures (eg, shivering) to increase the body temperature to the newly set levels. Excessive fevers interfere with the metabolic processes, leading eventually to demise.

Fever-reducing agents

The enzyme, cyclooxygenase, is responsible for the production of PGE$_2$ via the substrate, arachidonic acid, that is released from injured cell membranes. The production of PGE$_2$ is essential for fever. Hence, inhibitors of cyclooxygenase are potent antipyretics (ie, nonsteroidal anti-inflammatory drugs). Acetaminophen, which has minimal anti-inflammatory characteristics, is oxidized in the brain by the p450 cytochrome system. This oxidized form inhibits cyclooxygenase activity, also giving it antipyretic activity. There is no difference between oral aspirin and acetaminophen in reducing fever in humans. Corticosteriods, which inhibit the activity of phospholipase A$_2$ needed for the release of arachidonic acid from the membrane, also diminish the production of PGE$_2$ and, hence, have antipyretic properties [4]. Postoperative fevers can be suppressed with these agents to minimize patient discomfort, physiologic stress, and metabolic demands of fever and shivering.

Box 1. Causes of postoperative fever

Infectious

Surgical site infection
Pneumonia (ventilator-associated
  and aspiration)
Urinary tract infection (UTI) (usually
  with an indwelling bladder catheter)
Intravascular catheter-associated
  infection
Antibiotic-associated diiarrhea
Sinusitis
Otitis media
Parotitis
Intra-abdominal abscess
Meningitis
Acalculous cholecystitis
Transfusion-associated viral infections
Foreign body infection (orthopedic
  hardware, endovascular devices
  [eg, prosthetic heart valves, grafts,
  and stents])
Osteomyelitis
Endocarditis

Noninfectious

Surgical site inflammation without
  infection
Hematoma or seroma
Suture reaction

Thrombosis
  DVT
  Pulmonary embolism (thrombotic or
    fat embolism)

Inflammatory
  Gout or pseudogrout
  Pancreatitis

Vascular
  Cerebral infarction or hemorrhage
  Subarachnoid hemorrhage
  Myocardial infarction
  Bowel ischemia or infarction

Other
  Drug or alcohol withdrawal
  Transfusion reactions
  Transplant rejection
  Hyperthyroidism (including
    thyroid storm)
  Hypoadrenalism
  Cancer or neoplastic fever

This is unlikely to mask a significant underlying pathologic condition. Further treatment depends on the cause of the fever.

Postoperative fever

The operational definition of fever proposed by a consensus conference on sepsis and inflammation is a body temperature above 38°C (100.4°F) [2]. Fever above 38°C is common in the first few days after major surgery. Most early postoperative fever is caused by the inflammatory stimulus of surgery and resolves spontaneously. Postoperative fevers also may be the result, however, of serious complications and a thorough differential diagnosis is essential. This must include infectious and noninfectious causes (Box 1) [5].

Fevers greater than 38°C (100.4°F) require investigation. Timing of the fever postoperatively is the most important factor in determining its cause. This usually is classified as immediate, acute (24–72 hours postoperatively), subacute (within the first week), or delayed.

Fevers within the first 24 hours

Immediate fever mostly is the result of medications or blood products that were used during the course of the surgery. It also may represent fever from infection before surgery or it may be the result of trauma from the surgery itself (these resolve in 2 or 3 days and are proportional to the duration and extensiveness of the surgery). Fevers as a result of drug reaction often manifest with a rash and because of the vasodilatation are accompanied by hypotension, which often can be helpful in diagnosis. Fever as a result of malignant hyperthermia usually results within 30 minutes of starting inhalation anesthesia (discussed later). Infections usually result in fevers

3 ot 5 days postoperatively. There are two exceptions: group A streptococcus and *Clostridium perfringens*, which can cause fulminant infection within a few hours after surgery [5].

Fevers as a result of drugs can be divided into five categories: those resulting from hypersensitivity reactions, those resulting from altered thermoregulatory mechanisms, those related directly to administration of the drug, those that are direct extensions of the pharmacologic action of the drug, and those that are idiosyncratic reactions (Box 2) [6].

Fevers resulting from drugs are diagnosed by exclusion. In the absence of other causes of postoperative fever, it is prudent to identify drugs that may be the cause of the fever. Even though few, there are some clinical signs that may assist in the diagnosis. Presentation of drug fever sometimes can be accompanied by a rash (18%) [6]. In 20% of cases, there is an elevation of white cell count. Timing, alternatively, is not particularly helpful in making the diagnosis. The median time of onset is approximately 8 days and can vary from within 24 hours to many months. The pattern of fever also is not helpful, as it may vary from low-grade to high fever with chills and rigors. As with most fevers, there is an increase of 8 to 10 beats per minute with increase of 1° in temperature [6]. The only true way to make the diagnosis is to discontinue the drug or drugs. This should be performed in a sequential manner. Stopping all the drugs at once loses the opportunity to determine the specific drug responsible for the fever and also may put patients at unnecessary risk. Resolution of drug fever occurs within 72 to 96 hours. The most likely drug should be stopped first and so on. Rechallenge with the specific drug can confirm the result further if fever returns.

Immediate fevers also can be the result of transfusion reactions. If reaction is mild, no treatment is required. If reaction is characterized by tachycardia, chills, back pain, dyspnea, or microvascular bleeding, a major transfusion reaction should be assumed. In such instances, transfusions should be stopped and patients' blood crossmatched again. Should significant hemolysis occur, patients also require a forced diuresis and alkalization of the urine to prevent renal toxicity [7].

Box 2.

Antimicrobials
  Penicillins
  Cephalosporins
  Fluoroquinolones
  Vancomycin
  Sulfonamides
  Nitrofurantoin
  Rifampin
  Amphotericin B
Cardiovascular medications
  Thiazide diuretics
  Furosemide
  Spironolactone
  Hydralazine
  Quinidine
  Procainamide
  Alpha-methyldopa
Anticonvulsants
  Phenytoin
Other
  Heparin (especially unfractionated)
  Salicylates
  Nonsteroidal anti-inflammatory drugs
  Allopurinol
  Immunoglobulins
  Iodides
  Propylthiouracil
  Hydroxyurea

Mycophenolate mofetil

Fevers within 24 to 72 hours after surgery

Acute fevers are defined as those arising within the first week of surgery. There are many causes, including surgical site infection, intravascular catheters, aspiration pneumonia, pulmonary embolism, and UTI.

Atelectasis is considered a common cause of early postoperative fever. No correlation exists to date, however, between the presence of atelectasis and the appearance of fever. At best, the data show atelectasis is a 56% accurate predictor of postoperative fever [5]. This is close to coincidental. Most fevers credited to atelectasis resolve within 2 to 3 days. An argument can be made that these fevers are the result of surgical trauma itself. The mechanism by which fever is believed to develop from atelectasis centers around the imperfect expansion of certain areas of the lung. Mainly during prolonged procedures with the use of endotracheal tubes and because of mucus retained in the airways, obstruction occurs in the distal bronchial segments. The affected segments collapse when the air is absorbed. Breakdown of tissues in these areas or invasion by bacterial organisms can launch a cytokine-mediated febrile response. Current therapy for mild atelectasis entails deep breathing exercises (ie, incentive spirometry) and ambulation. Severe symptoms accompanied by spiking fevers and dyspnea may need radiographic assessment to rule out large segment collapse and exclude pneumonia [7].

Another pulmonary event that may result in fever in acute fever is thromboembolism. The most common cause of such an event is deep vein thrombosis (DVT), which shoots projectiles into the lung field. Pulmonary embolism can be accompanied by chest pain and dyspnea. Often, DVT is silent (50%–70%); hence, a negative leg examination cannot be used to rule out thromboembolism. When positive, signs of DVT, include swelling and pain of the affected area. Homans' sign refers to the presence of pain in the calf on forced dorsiflexion. This method of diagnosis has gone out of favor because of its low sensitivity and the speculation that this maneuver actually may dislodge the clot precipitating a thromboembolic event. If thromboembolism is suspected, there is a protocol for diagnosis and treatment that can be used; the details are beyond the scope of this article. Ventilation perfusion scans and pulmonary angiography are useful in the diagnosis. Ultrasound imaging and impedance plethysmography have a 90% accuracy in identifying DVT. Treatment of DVT is based on systemic anticoagulation. Five to 10 days of bed rest usually precede DVT. Oral and maxillofacial surgery patients begin ambulating relatively quickly, making thromboembolism a rare occurrence.

More commonly, fever may result from aspiration pneumonia. In the presence of a depressed cough reflex, aspiration after general anesthesia is a worrisome complication. This risk is increased in patients in intermaxillary fixation. Pneumonia from aspiration of foreign material is manifested more commonly in the right lung. Fever from this can be evident 3 to 5 days later or up to 2 to 3 weeks after surgery. A radiograph often can make the diagnosis. Chest radiograph findings in patients are characterized by the presence of infiltrates, predominantly the alveolar type, in one or both lower lobes or diffuse simulation of the appearance of pulmonary edema. Volume loss in any lobar area suggests obstruction (eg, by aspirated particles or other foreign bodies) in the bronchus. Treatment is based on radiographic findings and blood counts. Management by a specialist usually begins with broad-spectrum antibiotics [7].

UTIs also are high up on the differential in fevers during the acute phase (within the first week of surgery), occurring mainly in patients who have indwelling urethral catheters. The probability of a UTI increases with the duration of catheterization. UTI is more common in patients who have undergone a genitourinary procedure and in those who have chronic, indwelling catheters before surgery. Women are at greater risk for this type of infection because they have a shorter urethra than in males. Symptoms that may occur in conjunction are dysuria, burning on urination, and cloudy urine. Urinalysis and a culture are part of the work-up and antibiotic therapy is the appropriate treatment [7].

Another common site for infections is the intravenous (IV) catheter. Symptoms of phlebitis include pain, edema, erythema, and streaking on the limb. Treatment is with anti-inflammatories and heat packs to the site. IV sites are suspect if in place for longer than 24 hours. All lines should be restarted in a new location every 72 hours.

The surgical site itself can be the source of infection, resulting in fever. This can manifest as early as 3 days after surgery but is seen more commonly a week or more after the procedure when the patient already is discharged. Examination of the site shows swelling, erythema, pain, discharge, and possible dehiscence. The presence of pus is an indication to open the wound. Cultures should determine antibiotic coverage.

Malignant hyperthermia and subacute bacterial endocarditis

Malignant hyperthermia is a rare genetic disorder occurring with a prevalence of 1 in 50,000 adults. It occurs in approximately 1 in 15,000 episodes of general anesthesia and can be precipitated by any of the inhalational anesthetics (eg, halothane) and succinylcholine. The onset usually is within an hour after administration of the anesthetic but can be delayed up to 10 hours after induction. The mechanism is an uncontrolled efflux of calcium from the sarcoplasmic reticulum with subsequent tetany, increased skeletal metabolism, and heat production, with the earliest finding presenting as an increase in the end-tidal carbon dioxide. Muscle rigidity (especially masseter stiffness), sinus tachycardia, and skin cyanosis follow and significant hyperthermia (45°C) occurs minutes to hours later. The core body temperature tends to rise 1°C every 5 to 60 minutes. Dantrolene is the mainstay of treatment and should be initiated as soon as the diagnosis is suspected. Dantrolene is a nonspecific skeletal muscle relaxant that acts by

Box 3. Evaluation of patients who have postoperative fever

History

Review record for
  Preoperative course and presentation
  Operation (emergent or elective, intraoperative complications)
  Postoperative course
  Past medical history and underlying medical problems
  Allergies
  Medications
  Location of catheters and time of placement

Ask nursing staff about
  Sputum amount and quality
  Diarrhea
  Any areas of skin breakdown or rashes

Ask patients about
  Cough
  Pain

Laboratory[a]

  Urinalysis and culture
  Sputum gram stain and culture
  Blood culture (from catheters and peripherally—minimum of two)
  Wound culture
  Complete blood count with differential
  Chest radiograph
  Additional blood or radiographic studies might be indicated by specific findings. As examples, abdominal pain might indicate the need for blood tests for hepatic and pancreatic enzymes or abdominal CT scanning; unilateral leg edema might indicate the need for ultrasound to rule out DVT.

Physical examination

  Review records for vital signs. Determine range in the past day and peak daily values during hospital stay. Check nurses' notes for fevers not recorded in the vital signs chart.
  Temperature
  Heart rate
  Respiratory rate

Examine
  Skin for rash, ecchymoses, injection site eryethema, and hematoma
  Lungs
  Heart for tachycardia or new murmur
  Abdomen for tenderness, bloating, and bowel sounds
  Operative site and lymphatic drainage
  Catheter entry sties
  Lower legs for evidence of DVT

[a] Studies should be ordered based on patient evaluation; no test is mandatory.

---

blocking the release of calcium from the sarcoplasmic reticulum. The drug is most effective when given early in the illness when maximal calcium can be retained within the sarcoplasmic reticulum. A 2-mg/kg IV bolus is given and should be repeated every 5 minutes until symptoms abate up to a maximum dose of 10 mg/kg. This may be repeated every 10 to 15 hours. After initial response, the drug should be continued orally, at a dose of 4 to 8 mg/kg/d, in four divided does, for 3 days [8].

Subacute bacterial endocarditis (SBE) can be a diagnostic challenge; however, patients at high risk are identified easily, as they report of history of valvular damage. The diagnosis of SBE is suggested by a history of an indolent process characterized by fever, fatigue, anorexia, back pain, and weight loss. Less common developments are a cerebrovascular accident or congestive heart failure. The condition may manifest in the delayed postoperative period. Most subacute disease caused by *Streptococci viridans* is related to dental disease; however, most cases are not caused by dental procedures but by transient bacteremias arising from gingivitis. In 85% of patients, symptoms of endocarditis appear within 2 weeks of dental or other procedures. The interval between the onset of disease and diagnosis averages approximately 6 weeks. The fact that less than 50% of patients have previously diagnosed underlying valvular disease significantly limits the effectiveness of antibiotic prophylaxis. Once identified, treatment is with long-term IV antibiotics [9].

Fever work-up

Because of the variety of causes of postoperative fever, a work-up must involve a logical sequence of diagnostic tests and studies to narrow the list and eventually pinpoint the cause. Chest radiography, urinalysis, and blood and urine cultures are not indicated for all postoperative patients who have fever. The need for laboratory testing should be determined by the findings of a careful history and physical examination. A systematic examination sequence is depicted in Box 3 [3], based on the timing of onset of fever and the many possible causes. The work-up should include inspection (of wound sites, catheters, drains, and so forth), physical examination (specifically pulmonary, cardiac, and abdominal), and measurement of calf diameter to rule out possible DVT. Cultures should include blood from at least two sites, clean catch urine, and any drainage from the wound. A chest radiograph also is necessary to rule out pulmonary causes.

Treatment

Treatment of the fever is based first on an accurate diagnosis and then on discontinuation of the causative agent. Antimicrobial therapy is begun if the fever is of microbial origin. Dantrolene is used if malignant hyperthermia is suspected. Initial control of the temperature can be achieved by means of antipyretic agents (ie, acetaminophen or ibuprofen) to control the physiologic effects on the body of elevated temperatures. This should be followed by thorough physical examination and any necessary laboratory and diagnostic studies to eventually determine the cause.

References

[1] Mackowiak PA, Wasserman SS, Levine MM. A critical appraisal of 98.6 degrees F, the upper limit of the normal body temperature, and other legacies of Carl Reinhold August Wunderlich. JAMA 1992;268:1578–80.
[2] Marino P. Febrile patient. In: Marino P, editor. The ICU book. Baltimore: Williams & Wilkins; 1998. p. 485–501.
[3] August M. Postoperative care. In: Donoff RB, editor. Manual of oral and maxillofacial surgery. 2nd ed. St. Louis: Mosby; 1997. p. 161–7.
[4] Porat R, Charles D. Pathophysiology and treatment of fever in adults. In: Uptodate patient information, version 13.1. Available at: http://www.patients.update.com. Accessed March 2005.
[5] Weed H, Baddour L. Postoperative fever. In: Uptodate patient information, version 13.1. Available at: http://www.patients.update.com. Accessed March 2005.
[6] McDonald M, Sexton D. Drug fever. In: Uptodate patient information, version 13.1. Available at: http://www.patients.update.com. Accessed March 2005.
[7] Kwon P, Laskin D. Postoperative problems. In: Kwon P, Laskin D, editors. Clinician's manual of oral and maxillofacial surgery. 3rd ed. Hanover Park (IL): Quintessence Publishing; 2001. p. 263–7.
[8] Mechem C. Sever hyperthermia: heat stroke; neuroleptic malignant syndrome; and malignant hyperthermia. In: Uptodate patient information, version 13.1.
[9] Lawrence Jr P. Infective endocarditis. In: Emedicine articles. 2004. Available at: http://emedicine.com. Accessed March 2005.

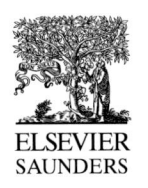

Perioperative Management of Patients Who Have Pulmonary Disease

Rana Y. Ali, MD[a,*], M. Scott Reminick, MD[a,b]

[a]*Division of Pulmonary and Critical Care Medicine, Department of Internal Medicine, The Brooklyn Hospital Center, Brooklyn, NY, USA*
[b]*College of Medicine, State University of New York, Downstate Medical Center, Brooklyn, NY, USA*

Patients who have pulmonary disease present a unique combination of problems to health care providers in the perioperative period. Although preoperative assessment of pulmonary function is a major consideration in patients who undergo a surgical procedure involving the chest and upper abdomen, a thorough assessment of patients who have underlying pulmonary disease helps to minimize the risk for perioperative complications in those undergoing any surgical procedure.

Rarely does the most severe of pulmonary disease exclude patients from a needed surgical procedure. Once patients are identified as at increased risk because of a pre-existing pulmonary condition, appropriate measures can be used to optimize patients' respiratory status and minimize the risk for postoperative pulmonary complications (PPCs). The complications range from minor atelectasis, dyspnea, cough, and increased sputum production to severe pneumonia and respiratory failure requiring prolonged mechanical ventilation. PPCs can have a serious impact on morbidity and mortality and can prolong a hospital stay by an average of 1 to 2 weeks [1,2]. The ability to predict accurately the risk for PPCs remains imprecise.

The purpose of preoperative pulmonary assessment is to predict which patients are at greatest risk for pulmonary complications and to determine which measures need to be taken to optimize the pulmonary status before surgery and minimize the risk to patients.

Preoperative assessment of risk

Risk factors include those that may be related to the underlying condition of patients or to a procedure itself. A thorough history and physical examination are the most valuable steps in identifying those at a higher risk for developing postoperative complications. A history of cough, dyspnea on exertion, wheezing, sputum production, and decreased exercise tolerance, along with pertinent physical findings, give clues to patients' underlying cardiopulmonary status. Further testing subsequently may be indicated to determine the extent of pulmonary compromise.

Preoperative pulmonary function testing

Routine use of pulmonary function testing is not indicated. Simple spirometry is done if patients have evidence of underlying pulmonary disease from history, physical examination, or chest radiograph or if they have a history of smoking. Although pulmonary function testing and arterial blood gases are useful in predicting pulmonary function after lung resection, they do not predict PPCs [3].

Patients having low-risk surgery do not need preoperative pulmonary function testing. In those patients who have advanced age, known pulmonary

---

* Corresponding author. Division of Pulmonary and Critical Care Medicine, The Brooklyn Hospital Center, 121 DeKalb Avenue, Brooklyn, NY 11201.

1042-3699/06/$ – see front matter © 2005 Elsevier Inc. All rights reserved.
doi:10.1016/j.coms.2005.09.009

oralmaxsurgery.theclinics.com

disease, or anticipated prolonged anesthesia time, however, knowledge of spirometry data can assist in optimization of preoperative and postoperative care [4].

Upper abdominal surgery and thoracotomy are associated with a higher incidence of PPCs; therefore, it is prudent to know of any underlying lung dysfunction before surgery. With the exception of lung resection, surgery should not be denied based on pulmonary function testing alone.

A recent study reviewing patients who had chronic obstructive pulmonary disease (COPD) and were undergoing high-risk surgery did not show spirometry as an independent predictor of PPCs. Those patients who developed serious complications postoperatively, however, had a greater severity of disease based on spirometry [5].

In patients undergoing lung resection who have severe obstructive lung disease with a forced expiratory volume in 1 second (FEV_1) less than 0.8 L/s (less than 30% of predicted in a normal adult male), there is a significant increase in morbidity and mortality postoperatively. A FEV_1 of less than 0.8 L/s is associated with the development of hypercapnia (arterial carbon dioxide tension [$PaCO_2$] >45 mm Hg) [6]. Diffusion capacity of carbon monoxide (DLCO) is a measure of the integrity of the alveolar membrane and a good predictor of postoperative morbidity and mortality. A DLCO less than 40% associated with a borderline FEV_1 is a cause of higher mortality [7].

Arterial blood gas analysis is not done routinely. It is required if significant lung dysfunction is suspected. Arterial carbon dioxide tension ($PaCO_2$) of more than 45 mm Hg indicates significant alveolar hypoventilation and chronic respiratory failure and is known to be associated with increased respiratory complications [8]. Subsequent studies show that patients who have a $PaCO_2$ greater than 45 mm Hg do well postoperatively and that elevated carbon dioxide is not predictive of PPCs [9]. Preoperative arterial blood gas values serve as a baseline and aid in ventilatory management in the postoperative period. Low-resting PaO_2 is not a strong predictor of PPC [8].

Risk factors for developing postoperative pulmonary complications

Patient-related risk factors
Smoking. Smoking is identified as a major risk factor for PPCs. This first was reported in 1944 [10] and since then several studies have supported this.

Studies show that risk declines after 8 weeks of cessation of smoking before surgery [11]. Patients in need of an urgent surgical procedure should quit smoking for as long as possible before surgery, even if it is only for 24 hours, to decrease the cardiac effects of nicotine and reduce carbon monoxide levels (Box 1) [12,13].

Underlying lung conditions. Chronic obstructive pulmonary disease and asthma. In patients who have COPD and asthma, optimal reduction of symptoms should be sought aggressively before a surgical procedure. If an acute exacerbation is present, elective surgery should be postponed until airflow obstruction is optimized adequately with medications. A combination of medications, smoking cessation, and physical therapy reduces the risk for PPCs [14,15].

Obstructive sleep apnea. Obstructive sleep apnea (OSA) may be secondary to disproportionate anatomy of the upper airways [16,17]. The site of obstruction can be at the level of nose, soft palate, or base of the tongue [18]. Corrective surgery is indicated in some patients who have OSA; however, the rate of complications arising from airway compromise may be increased. Surgically induced upper airway edema and the effects of sedatives and other anesthetic agents that decrease the muscle tone and alter the pattern of breathing accentuate airway compromise [19].

Box 1. Risk factors for developing postoperative pulmonary complications

Patient-related risk factors

1. Smoking
2. Underlying lung condition
3. General health status
4. Age
5. Obesity

Procedure-related risk factors

1. Site of surgery
2. Type of surgery—open versus laparoscopic
3. Duration of surgical procedure
4. Type of anesthesia

Pulmonary hypertension. The adrenergic response to surgical stimulation and the circulatory effects of anesthetic agents, endotracheal intubation, positive pressure ventilation, blood loss, fluid shifts, and alterations in body temperature impose an additional burden on an already compromised cardiovascular system. Preoperative pulmonary hypertension is a significant and independent predictor of hospital mortality in elderly patients undergoing cardiac procedures [20]. Similarly, in pregnant women, pulmonary hypertension carries a high risk for maternal death, approximately 30% to 50% [21]. Finally, in a retrospective study, patients who had moderate to severe portopulmonary hypertension (mean pulmonary artery pressure greater than 35 mm Hg) and underwent liver transplantation had a mortality of up to 50% [22].

In patients who have severe pulmonary hypertension and a cardiac shunt, systemic hypotension results in an increased right-to-left shunt and predisposes patients to the development of acidosis, which can lead to further decreases in systemic vascular resistance. Pulmonary vascular resistance may be increased by hypoxia, hypercapnia, endogenous catecholamines (as a result of stress or pain), or Valsalva maneuvers. Avoidance of these risk factors is essential in minimizing perioperative complications. Intraoperative hemodynamic monitoring using pulmonary artery catheterization often is used. The underlying cause of secondary pulmonary hypertension must be treated before surgery. Patients' functional status should be optimized before surgery to reduce the perioperative mortality.

General health status. The Goldman Cardiac Index and the American Society of Anesthesiologists Classification evaluate the risk for overall perioperative mortality and are strongly predictive of PPCs [23–25]. Poor exercise tolerance identifies patients at risk. In a study of patients 65 years or older, inability to perform 2 minutes of supine bicycle exercise sufficient to raise the heart rate to 99 beats per minute is the strongest predictor of pulmonary complications [26].

Age. Age by itself is not found to be an independent predictor of PPCs [27]. Older patients may have accompanying lung disease or cardiac disease predisposing them to ventilatory failure.

Obesity. Several studies looking at risk factors for pulmonary complications do not find obesity independently associated with PPCs [28,29]. In patients who have OSA, a condition commonly associated with obesity, however, the risk for cardiopulmonary complication, such as upper airway obstruction, oxygen desaturation, and cardiorespiratory arrest, increases [19].

Procedure-related risk factors
Site of the surgical procedure. This is a strong predictor of postoperative complications. Risk increases as the incision approaches the diaphragm [30,31]. Thoracic and upper abdominal surgery carries the highest risk (10%–40%). The risk of pulmonary complications is much lower in laparoscopic cholecystectomy (0.3%–0.4%) compared with open cholecystectomy (13%–33%) [32,33].

The duration of surgery. Procedures lasting more than 3 hours are associated with a higher risk for pulmonary complications [34].

Type of anesthesia. Compared with general anesthesia, the reported risk for pulmonary complications is much lower with epidural or spinal anesthesia [15].

Patients receiving long-acting neuromuscular blockers, such as pancuronium, are at a higher risk for developing pulmonary complications compared with those receiving shorter-acting or intermediate-acting agents, such as atracurium or vecuronium [35].

Perioperative pulmonary complication

Pathophysiology

The risk for developing pulmonary insufficiency postoperatively ranges from 5% to 80% [36]. During the postoperative period, the lungs are extremely vulnerable. Ventilation and perfusion are affected by anesthesia and tissue injury suffered as the result of the operative procedure.

Ventilation

The ventilatory pattern differs during the postoperative period. These changes depend on type of anesthesia, duration and type of surgery, pre-existing pulmonary status, and postoperative course of patients. Factors that affect ventilation during the postoperative period include

1. Low tidal volume leading to alveolar collapse and development of atelectasis
2. Decrease in residual volume, functional residual capacity, and vital capacity
3. Reduced lung compliance

4. Postoperative hypoxemia resulting from shunting and atelectasis

Postoperatively, patients lack the normal pattern of spontaneous deep breaths. This could be secondary to pain, narcotics, or anesthetic agents [37]. If spontaneous deep breaths to maximal lung inflation are eliminated from the pattern of breathing, alveolar collapse begins within 1 hour and progresses rapidly to produce significant transpulmonary shunting [37]. Maximal inflation deep breathing exercises at regular intervals help in returning the postoperative lung function toward normal [38].

In the recumbent position, superior lobes of the lungs are ventilated, whereas perfusion is preferential to the dependent lobes leading to shunting of blood, which results in hypoxemia. With time, lower lobe alveoli begin to collapse, leading to further atelectasis and hypoxemia. In patients who have underlying lung conditions, such as COPD, postoperative ventilatory problems may be accentuated.

Changes in the pulmonary interstitium

The pulmonary vascular bed is vulnerable to injury during and after surgery because of factors that include

1. Aggressive fluid resuscitation leading to increased hydrostatic pressure
2. Injury to the capillary membrane as a result of endotoxins released from tissue injury and microemboli
3. Left ventricular dysfunction with a resultant increase in left atrial pressure leading to transcapillary transudation
4. Poor nutrition with loss of proteins resulting in low oncotic pressure

Increase in hydrostatic pressure, decrease in oncotic pressure, and increase in capillary permeability may lead to the accumulation of fluid in the pulmonary interstitium and the alveolar space, decreasing lung compliance. This can cause atelectasis in the dependent portion of the lungs [39]. Not only does this affect gas exchange leading to hypoxemia but also atelectatic lung with inspissated secretions provide a breeding ground for bacteria making patients more prone to pulmonary infections postoperatively.

Effect of anesthesia on respiration

The status of the respiratory system can be affected by the anesthetic agent and instrumentation required during administration of anesthesia. Tracheal intubation and inhalation gases impair mucociliary transport, resulting in an increase in secretions. This may persist for 2 to 6 days postoperatively [40,41]. Endotracheal intubation also can cause bronchospasm by reflex stimulation of the airways. Prolonged anesthesia and surgery impair the function of lung inflammatory cells. A study by Kotani and coworkers shows that anesthetic agents (isoflurane and propofol) modulate alveolar macrophage function intraoperatively [42]. This may increase susceptibility to infection.

Anesthesia suppresses the normal cough reflex and glottic closure, thereby increasing the risk for aspiration. It also has a depressant effect on the central respiratory control center. Inhaled anesthetics result in rapid shallow breathing leading to a reduction in minute ventilation [43]. Anesthesia also decreases ventilatory response to hypercapnea and hypoxemia [44].

The volatile anesthetic agents shift the carbon dioxide curve to the right and depress the slope in a dose-dependent manner [44,45], whereas surgical stimulation produces an increase in minute ventilation and, thereby, reduces carbon dioxide (Fig. 1).

There also is a profound reduction in the ventilatory response to hypoxemia resulting from the use of inhaled anesthetics [45]. Agents, such as morphine, decrease hypoxic and hypercapnic ventilatory response [46]; propofol decreases ventilatory response to carbon dioxide [47] and produces apnea at induction doses. Ketamine has little effect on resting ventilation [44].

Patients who have COPD are more sensitive to the ventilatory depressant effects of the anesthetic agents; hence, the risk for hypercarbia and respiratory insufficiency increases [48]. Volatile anesthetic agents may cause a prolonged depression of hypoxic ventilatory drive well into the postoperative period. Most of these agents are metabolized slowly and are stored in the tissues (muscles and fat) from which they are released slowly during the recovery period and eliminated via the lungs. Patients who are dependent on the hypoxic ventilatory drive are at a risk for developing respiratory insufficiency even during the postoperative period [44].

Lung mechanics also are changed during anesthesia. With the induction of anesthesia, the diaphragm moves cranially, decreasing thoracic volume by approximately 0.5 liters [49,50]. Chest wall relaxation leads to a decrease in the transverse rib cage diameter, decreasing the thoracic volume even further (0.25 L) [50].

Loss of diaphragm tone and its movement cranially leads to development of areas of atelectasis

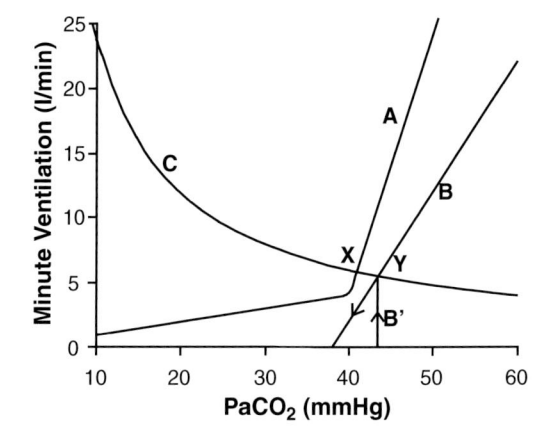

Fig. 1. Curve A represents the normal carbon dioxide response of an awake individual; the hockey stick appearance at low values of $PaCO_2$ corresponds to the observation that after hyperventilation, awake individuals do not become apneic but show a modest decrease in VE until $PaCO_2$ returns to its resting value. Curve B represents the carbon dioxide response curve after administration of a sedative or anesthetic medication, which decreases its slope by 50%. Note that the curve no longer has a hockey stick shape but falls linearly to a VE of 0 (the apneic threshold). Once apnea develops, the PCO_2 must increase to approximately the resting value before ventilation restarts, accounting for the hysteresis loop (line B). Curve C represents the carbon dioxide excretion hyperbola, which depends on the principle of conservation of mass: assuming constant carbon dioxide production, increasing VE decreases $PaCO_2$, whereas decreasing VE tends to increase $PaCO_2$. In the awake state, point X (the intersection of carbon dioxide response curve A with carbon dioxide excretion hyperbola C) defines the resting $PaCO_2$ and VE, whereas point Y represents the values of $PaCO_2$ and VE during sedation or anesthesia. (*From* Gross JB. When you breathe IN you inspire, when you DON'T breathe, you...expire. Anesthesiology 2003;99:767–70; with permission.)

[51]. In studies of patients under general anesthesia, CT scans of the chest demonstrate the appearance of crescent-shaped densities within approximately 5 minutes after induction of anesthesia, likely the result of compression atelectasis [52,53]. Patients who have COPD develop minimal or no atelectasis, probably because they develop airway closure before alveolar collapse [51].

With the induction of anesthesia, there is more ventilation to the nondependent areas of the lung, increasing the alveolar dead space and leading to an increase in ventilation perfusion mismatch [54]. Shunting of blood as a result of ventilation perfusion mismatch is accentuated by areas of atelectasis that develop during induction of anesthesia and is responsible for impairment of arterial oxygenation [55,56].

Postoperative pulmonary complications

Pulmonary complications may occur during the postoperative period and affect patients' clinical course adversely. Such complications include

1. Exacerbation of COPD or asthma
2. Hypoxemia
3. Aspiration
4. Atelectasis
5. Upper airway obstruction
6. Postobstructive pulmonary edema
7. Pneumonia
8. Pleural effusion
9. Pulmonary embolism
10. Tracheal lacerations or rupture
11. Bronchospasm

Exacerbation of asthma and chronic obstructive pulmonary disease

Patients who have well-controlled asthma need no further testing and present no additional risk for the development of PPCs. If the peak expiratory flow rate is less than 80% of predicted, use of systemic steroids during the perioperative period is recommended. Wheezing should be controlled with the use of inhaled β-agonists. The National Asthma Education and Prevention Program recommends use of systemic steroids during the perioperative period in patients who have wheezing, cough, chest tightness, or shortness of breath while they are on their usual outpatient therapy [57].

Corticosteroids in the perioperative period are demonstrated to be safe. They are not shown to cause an increase in the incidence of infection postoperatively [58]. Patients treated chronically with prednisone in doses of 20 mg daily for more than 3 weeks in the previous 6 months may exhibit suppression of adrenal hypothalamic axis and may require a maintenance dose. Those on 5-mg daily or less of prednisone should not have suppression and steroids may be discontinued as indicated.

Patients who have COPD must be treated aggressively to achieve their best baseline functional status before subjecting them to elective surgery. Use of inhaled β-agonists and anticholinergics helps with symptomatic improvement. A favorable outcome with reduction of postoperative complications is seen in patients treated with a combination of bronchodilators, antibiotics, systemic steroids, and chest physical therapy [14,59]. The role of smoking cessation is discussed elsewhere in this article.

Hypoxemia

Postoperative hypoxemia is defined as an arterial oxygen saturation of less than 90% or PaO$_2$ of less than 75% of the preoperative value [60]. It is more common after thoracic and abdominal surgeries [61]. Falls in arterial oxygen can range from as high as 20% to 30% in thoracic and abdominal surgery compared with 5% to 10% in nonthoracic surgeries [60]. Postoperative hypoxemia usually occurs during the first 48 hours but can persist for 4 to 5 days [62].

Factors contributing to the development of hypoxemia include anesthesia-induced hypoventilation and the loss of upper airway muscle tone, volume overload, inability to clear secretions, upper airway edema, aspiration, pulmonary embolism, and intrinsic lung conditions, such as an exacerbation of COPD and asthma.

The use of supplemental oxygen and identification of the underlying etiology are the primary goals of treatment. Patients' oxygen level should be maintained at a minimum PO$_2$ of 60 mm Hg or an oxygen saturation of 90%. Treatment should be directed to correct the underlying cause. Patients who have impending respiratory failure can be treated with noninvasive positive pressure ventilation, as this may improve lung volumes and facilitate gas exchange [63]. Refractory hypoxemia should be treated by intubation and mechanical ventilation.

Aspiration

Aspiration is a common complication, particularly during the course of general anesthesia. Endosseous implants used in oral and maxillofacial surgery can be aspirated intraoperatively and could be life threatening [64].

Conditions that predispose to aspiration include

- Reduced consciousness, resulting in compromise of the cough reflex and glottic closure
- Neurologic defects, resulting in dysphagia
- Surgery involving the upper airways, esophageal disorders, and gastric reflux
- Mechanical disruption of the normal anatomy of the glottis as a result of tracheostomy, endotracheal intubation, and nasogastric feeding
- Local pharyngeal anesthesia given during procedures like bronchoscopy and upper endoscopy
- Feeding gastrostomy [65]
- Recumbent position [66]

Risk factors for aspiration include advanced age, type of anesthesia, type of surgery (most common in cases of esophageal, upper abdominal, or emergency surgery), whether or not patients have had a recent meal, delayed gastric emptying or decreased lower esophageal sphincter tone, pregnancy, morbid obesity, and neuromuscular disorders.

Complications from aspiration range from chemical pneumonitis after aspiration of gastric contents [67] to a more fulminant adult respiratory distress syndrome (ARDS) [68]. Aspiration pneumonia results from infection caused by the bacteria that colonize the upper airway. Patients present later with complications characterized by suppuration and necrosis [69].

Elevation of the head of the bed to use gravity to prevent reflux and aspiration of gastric contents is of paramount importance [66].

Atelectasis

Development of atelectasis is the most common problem encountered during the postoperative period. Changes in lung mechanics during anesthesia and surgery contribute significantly to the development of atelectasis. Primary prevention is the mainstay of treatment. Lung expansion maneuvers, adequate pain control, and pulmonary toileting are some of the measures that should be taken to avoid the development of atelectasis. Bronchoscopy for extraction of secretions in patients who have atelectasis has limited efficacy [70,71]. Use of mucolytic agents, such as N-acetylcysteine, neither decreases sputum production nor the incidence of atelectasis or pneumonia [72,73] and may induce bronchospasm.

Upper airway obstruction

Postoperative stridor may occur in the recovery phase and should be addressed immediately. Acute upper airway obstruction can be caused by laryngospasm, laryngeal edema, or mechanical obstruction from the tongue or oropharyngeal soft tissue. It is a true emergency that may warrant intubation. Inhaled racemic epinephrine and steroids may be of benefit. Bronchodilators, systemic steroids, and Heliox may provide temporary support until definitive intervention can be provided [74,75].

Postobstructive pulmonary edema

Also known as negative pressure pulmonary edema, postobstructive pulmonary edema is a known but rare complication during the postoperative period, resulting from laryngospasm or other forms of upper airway obstruction [76,77]. The etiology of negative pressure pulmonary edema is related to the generation of markedly negative intrathoracic pressure resulting from forced inspiration against a closed glottis, referred to as the Müller's (or reverse Valsalva's) maneuver. This results in transudation of fluid from pulmonary capillaries into the interstitium after relief of the upper airway obstruction [77,78].

Factors that might contribute to the development of upper airway obstruction include obesity, short neck or larger neck circumference, history of OSA, and prior ear, nose, and throat surgery. Laryngospasm-induced pulmonary edema also is reported in young athletic adults who have no other risk factors [79].

Development of edema normally occurs immediately after relief of obstruction; however, it can be delayed for several hours [78]. Longer monitoring, therefore, is recommended in patients who develop laryngospasm in the postoperative period [78,80].

Treatment mainly is supportive. Maintenance of a patent airway and adequate oxygenation is important. Recovery normally occurs in a short period of time. Some cases require intubation and mechanical ventilation [78]. The role of diuretics and steroids remain controversial [78–81].

Pneumonia

Patients are at increased risk for aspiration in the postoperative period for reasons discussed previously. Aspiration of acidic gastric content as a result of regurgitation or vomiting can result in the development of chemical pneumonitis. The presentation includes dyspnea, fever, tachycardia, wheezing, or cough. Infiltrates on chest radiograph usually appear within the first 24 hours. Most patients recover completely; however, some patients may develop ARDS or superimposed bacterial infection.

Intraoperative and immediate postoperative aspiration in patients receiving general anesthesia occur mostly during tracheal extubation and laryngoscopy. Poor general health of patients and emergency surgery are associated with a greater risk for aspiration [82].

Patients should be monitored closely for 24 to 48 hours for the development of pneumonitis. Adequacy of a patent airway should be maintained. Supplemental oxygen is needed in the setting of hypoxemia. In severe cases, mechanical ventilation may be needed. Prophylactic antibiotics are not recommended, as they may increase the incidence of colonization by resistant organisms.

Nosocomial, or hospital-acquired, pneumonia is defined as pneumonia occurring 48 hours after hospital admission in patients who do not have evidence of infection on admission [83]. Postoperative nosocomial pneumonia occurs mostly within the first 5 postoperative days. Common organisms include *Staphylococcus aureus* and gram-negative bacteria [84]. Infection with highly resistant organisms, such as *Pseudomonas aeruginosa*, *Acinetobacter* species, and methicillin-resistant *Staphylococcus aureus*, can affect the postoperative course adversely and be fatal. Treatment with broad-spectrum antibiotics is recommended until identification of the offending organism is made by blood or respiratory culture, at which time a focused antibiotic regimen may be used.

Pleural effusion

Large pleural effusions compromising ventilation should be drained before surgery. Small pleural effusions are encountered more commonly in patients after cardiothoracic or upper abdominal surgery. They typically resolve on their own within a few days. Effusions frequently are associated with atelectasis and resolve with adequate lung re-expansion.

Pulmonary embolism

Despite significant advances in the prevention and treatment of venous thromboembolism, pulmonary embolism remains the most common preventable cause of hospital death. Pulmonary embolism, if untreated, is associated with a mortality rate as high as 30%; however, this can be decreased significantly to as low as 2% to 8% with prompt diagnosis and adequate treatment with anticoagulation [85,86]. In patients undergoing elective general surgery who do not receive prophylaxis, the occurrence rate of fatal pulmonary embolism is 0.1% to 0.8%.

The Prospective Investigation of Pulmonary Embolism Diagnosis (PIOPED) study identified the following risk factors in the development of pulmonary embolism

- Immobilization
- Surgery within the last 3 months
- Stroke
- History of venous thromboembolism
- Malignancy

Autopsy studies show that 65% to 90% of pulmonary emboli arise from the lower extremities. The diagnosis is made by a thorough clinical assessment, lung scanning, and lower extremity Doppler studies.

Patients can present with signs and symptoms of dyspnea, pleuritic pain, cough, and hemoptysis. On physical examination, they may have tachypnea, rales, tachycardia, a fourth heart sound, and an accentuated pulmonic component of the second heart sound. Some patients can present with fever, generally less than 102°F, without any apparent cause of infection. The syndrome of pleuritic pain or hemoptysis without cardiovascular collapse is the most commonly recognized syndrome (65%); isolated dyspnea is observed in 22%. Circulatory collapse is uncommon (8%).

Simultaneous initiation of heparin (either unfractionated or low molecular weight) and oral warfarin is recommended in medically stable patients and should be overlapped for a minimum of 4 to 5 days until the international normalized ratio (INR) is in the therapeutic range (2.0 to 3.0) for 2 consecutive days [87].

The first thromboembolic event occurring in the setting of reversible risk factors (such as immobilization, surgery, trauma, or estrogen use) should be treated with warfarin therapy for 3 to 6 months [88,89]. In those patients who have a continuing risk factor that potentially is reversible (eg, prolonged bed rest), long-term therapy should be continued until the risk factor is reversed. IVC filter placement is recommended when anticoagulation is contraindicated or with recurrent thromboembolism despite adequate anticoagulation.

Fat embolism is a syndrome that typically manifests 24 to 72 hours after an initial insult, such as long bone fracture, orthopedic surgery, or soft tissue injury. Rarely, cases occur as early as 12 hours or as late as 2 weeks after the inciting event [90]. Affected patients present with a classic triad: hypoxemia, neurologic abnormalities, and a petechial rash. Overall mortality ranges from 5% to 15% across studies [91]. Treatment generally is supportive.

Tracheal laceration and perforation

These complications may be related directly to instrumentation. They can occur because of a difficult intubation [92]. Their presence can be detected immediately because of development of sudden respiratory compromise. Subcutaneous emphysema, pneumomediastinum, or pneumothorax may develop. In some cases, however, the presence of an endotracheal tube can mask their presentation until after extubation [93]. Their occurrence may be life threatening, requiring prompt surgical intervention.

Bronchospasm

Bronchospasm can be caused by reflex stimulation of the airways during instrumentation, aspiration, or histamine release caused by medications, such as morphine or atracurium. Treatment consists of removal of the irritant factor. Beta-2-sympathomimetic bronchodilators provide quick relief. If the cause is secondary to an inflammatory process, systemic steroids followed by inhaled steroids may be needed.

Risk reduction strategies

The goal of implementing perioperative pulmonary risk reduction strategies is to maintain the normal pattern of breathing and adequate inflation of the lungs (Box 2).

Preoperative preparation

Smoking cessation

The importance of smoking cessation cannot be stressed enough. Smoking preoperatively affects

---

Box 2. Strategies to reduce postoperative pulmonary complications

Preoperative

- Smoking cessation preferably 8 weeks before surgery
- Treatment of bronchospasm
- Optimization of airway obstruction in OSA
- Anticoagulation in venous thromboembolism (VTE)
- Treatment of upper respiratory tract infection
- Patient education
- Correction of electrolyte imbalance

Intraoperative

- Type of anesthesia: preferably spinal or epidural
- Shorten duration of operations to less than 3 hours
- Preferably laparoscopic surgeries
- Avoidance of long-acting neuromuscular blockers

Postoperative

- Lung expansion maneuvers
- Adequate pain control
- Deep vein thrombosis (DVT) prophylaxis
- Early ambulation

postoperative recovery. After surgery, smokers are more likely to

- Have pulmonary, circulatory, and infectious complications and impaired wound healing [94,95]
- Have reduced bone fusion
- Be admitted to an intensive care unit [96,97]
- Have increased risk for in-hospital mortality [96]

Before elective surgery, 8 weeks of abstinence from smoking decreases respiratory complications [98]. The potential benefits of preoperative smoking cessation counseling and nicotine replacement are demonstrated in a prospective, randomized trial of 120 smokers awaiting major orthopedic surgery [99]. Patients who underwent counseling and nicotine replacement 6 to 8 weeks before surgery had a lower rate of overall postoperative complications compared with patients in the control group (18% versus 52%).

One study of patients undergoing cardiac surgery shows that patients who had stopped smoking for less than 2 months before surgery had a higher incidence of PPCs [11]. This study also shows that patients who abstained from smoking for more than 6 months had a complication rate similar to patients who never smoked. Nevertheless, patients should stop smoking for as long as possible before surgery to decrease the carbon monoxide levels and the effect of nicotine on the heart.

Interventions for smoking cessation are effective in smokers making an attempt to quit. Individual behavioral support is effective in helping smokers quit for at least 6 months. An estimated 8% of smokers are successful with this approach [100]. Adding nicotine replacement therapy or bupropion to behavioral support increases 6-month success rates on average by 8% to 9% [101]. Studies show that 1 in 5 smokers who want to make an attempt to quit is successful if given appropriate therapy [102].

Obstructive lung disease

Well-controlled asthmatics have no additional risk for developing perioperative pulmonary complications. Patients should be continued on their normal maintenance therapy that consists typically of an inhaled steroid or long-acting bronchodilators. In patients who present with wheezing, aggressive therapy is required before surgery to control bronchospasm. In addition to bronchodilators, systemic corticosteroids are recommended for patients who are symptomatic (wheezing, chest tightness, and cough) or have FEV_1 of less than 80% of predicted.

Patients who have COPD are at a higher risk for developing respiratory complications and should be optimized adequately to achieve their best possible baseline function. A combination of bronchodilators, antibiotics, systemic steroids, and smoking cessation and chest physiotherapy decreases the rate of PPCs in patients presenting with an acute exacerbation of COPD [14,15]. Patients who continue to have symptoms despite bronchodilator therapy and have not reached their baseline lung function should be given a course of systemic steroids 2 weeks before surgery [103].

Patients presenting with chronic hypoxemia may have few if any symptoms referable to the decrease in oxygenation. Assessment of arterial blood gases or pulse oximetry, therefore, is the only reliable method for detecting hypoxemia. Arterial blood gas analysis also is helpful in assessing the presence and severity of hypercapnia, which can complicate oxygen therapy. In patients presenting with hypoxemia, supplemental oxygen should be supplied at the lowest level necessary to maintain a PO_2 of at least 60 mm Hg or an oxygen saturation of 90% or greater.

Obstructive sleep apnea

Patients who have diagnosed OSA by polysomnography are advised to use continuous positive airway pressure (CPAP). Nasal CPAP should be used for at least 2 weeks before surgery. Postsurgery CPAP is used even when patients are awake to decrease edema and prevent rapid eye movement rebound [104]. Analgesics and sedatives may interfere with the normal pattern of breathing and also increase upper airway resistance by decreasing muscle tone. They should be used cautiously. A temporary tracheotomy is considered in patients who have a difficult airway and significant craniofacial abnormalities. It is reserved for patients who have severe OSA in whom other medical and surgical treatments have failed.

Initial postoperative monitoring is recommended in the ICU to detect any sign of airway compromise or cardiac arrhythmias. Airway compromise can develop 36 hours after surgery [19]; hence, it is recommended that inspection of the airways by fiberoptic laryngoscopy be performed before discharge [105].

Venous thromboembolism

In patients who have DVT, surgery should be deferred, if possible, until patients have received at least 1 month, preferably 3 months, of anticoagulation. If surgery must be performed within 1 month of an acute VTE, intravenous unfractionated heparin should be administered while the INR is less than 2.0. If surgery must be performed within 2 weeks after an acute episode, intravenous heparin may be withheld 6 hours preoperatively and 12 hours postoperatively, if the surgery is short. If the acute event was within 2 weeks of major surgery or patients have a higher risk for postoperative bleeding, a vena caval filter should be inserted preoperatively or intraoperatively [106].

Warfarin should be withheld for only four doses if the most recent episode of VTE is between 1 and 3 months before surgery. If patients have been anticoagulated for 3 or more months, five doses of warfarin can be withheld before surgery [107].

Antibiotics

Preoperative antibiotic therapy is not indicated unless there is presence of pulmonary infection evident by purulent sputum or change in the character of sputum [59]. In patients who have stable COPD, antibiotics are not indicated unless there is presence of bronchiectasis or immune deficiency.

The risk for developing pulmonary complications in adults who have upper respiratory tract infection has not been studied; however, elective surgeries should be postponed in the presence of upper respiratory tract infection.

Patient education

Lung expansion maneuvers reduce the risk for developing atelectasis. The importance of teaching lung expansion maneuvers before surgery cannot be stressed enough. Preoperative education regarding lung expansion maneuvers reduces pulmonary complications more than instruction given after surgery [108,109]. Deep breathing exercises, chest physical therapy, and incentive spirometry consistently decrease the risk for PPCs [110].

Electrolyte imbalance

Abnormalities in electrolyte levels, such as phosphate and calcium, may interfere with the function of respiratory muscles, including the diaphragm, and should be corrected before surgery [111,112].

Intraoperative strategies

Type of anesthesia

Spinal or epidural anesthesia should be preferred, if possible, as general anesthesia is associated with a higher risk for PPCs [113]. Neuromuscular blockers should be avoided and, if used, intermediate-acting agents should be preferred over long-acting agents [35,114].

Type and duration of surgery

As a surgical incision approaches the diaphragm, the risk for PPCs increases. Thoracic and upper abdominal surgeries are associated with higher morbidity and mortality secondary to pulmonary complications. Surgical procedures lasting less than 3 hours are associated with lesser risk for developing PPCs [34].

Postoperative strategies

Lung expansion maneuvers

1. Deep breathing exercises, which are a part of chest physical therapy, improve lung volume after abdominal surgery and are recommended in the postoperative period [108].
2. Incentive spirometry prevents the development of atelectasis. Studies do not show a significant difference between incentive spirometry and chest physical therapy in reducing PPCs [108,115]. Use of incentive spirometry preoperatively, however, can give an idea of patients' baseline that can be used as a guide in the postoperative period.
3. Intermittent positive pressure breathing is not more effective than incentive spirometry or deep breathing exercises [108]. It causes significant abdominal distension. It is indicated in patients who have neuromuscular disorders in whom other modalities cannot be used.
4. CPAP is effort independent. It is found as effective as deep breathing exercises or incentive spirometry [116]. It also may be associated with complications, such as abdominal distension, patient discomfort, and barotrauma.

Pain control

Adequate pain control improves compliance with deep breathing and encourages early ambulation. Postoperative epidural analgesia is recommended after high-risk thoracic or upper abdominal procedures [117]. Intercostal nerve block is an option if epidural analgesia cannot be given [118].

Deep vein thrombosis prophylaxis

Pulmonary embolism can be a fatal complication during the postoperative period. DVT prophylaxis, using either low molecular weight heparin or warfarin, is recommended depending on the site and type of surgical procedure. If, for some reason, anticoagulation cannot be given, then pneumatic compression devices or compression stockings should be used [119].

Early ambulation

Early mobilization of patients decreases the incidence of venous thromboembolism and should be encouraged.

Summary

Perioperative pulmonary complications are a major cause of mortality and morbidity. In addition to the impact on patients' well being, an increased length of stay in the hospital results in an added economic burden on the health care system. Patients who have pulmonary disease must be assessed fully before surgery. A detailed history and thorough physical examination are key to perioperative assessment, and additional testing may not be necessary in all patients. Identification and optimization of risk factors can help reduce the complication rate. Strategies need to be used starting in the preoperative period and continuing through the postoperative period to minimize the risk for complications and expedite the recovery of patients.

References

[1] Lawrence VA, Dhanda R, Hilsenbeck SG, et al. Risk of pulmonary complications after elective abdominal surgery. Chest 1996;110:744–50.
[2] Lawrence VA, Hilsenbeck SG, Mulrow CD, et al. Incidence and hospital stay for cardiac and pulmonary complications after abdominal surgery. J Gen Intern Med 1995;10:671–8.
[3] Lawrence VA, Page CP, Harris GD. Preoperative spirometry before abdominal operations. A critical appraisal of its predictive value. Arch Intern Med 1989; 149:280–5.
[4] Wait J. Southwestern Internal Medicine Conference: preoperative pulmonary evaluation. Am J Med Sci 1995;310:118–25.
[5] Kroenke K, Lawrence VA, Theroux JF, et al. Postoperative complications after thoracic and major abdominal surgery in patients with and without obstructive lung disease. Chest 1993;104:1445–51.
[6] Segall JJ, Butterworth BA. Ventilatory capacity in chronic bronchitis in relation to carbon dioxide retention. Scand J Respir Dis 1966;47:215–24.
[7] Markos J, Mullan BP, Hillman DR, et al. Preoperative assessment as a predictor of mortality and morbidity after lung resection. Am Rev Respir Dis 1989;139: 902–10.
[8] Olsen GN, Block AJ, Swenson EW, et al. Pulmonary function evaluation of the lung resection candidate: a prospective study. Am Rev Respir Dis 1975;111: 379–87.
[9] Stephan F, Boucheseiche S, Hollande J, et al. Pulmonary complications following lung resection: a comprehensive analysis of incidence and possible risk factors. Chest 2000;118:1263–70.
[10] Morton H. Tobacco smoking and pulmonary complications after surgery. Lancet 1944;1:368–70.
[11] Warner MA, Offord KP, Warner ME, et al. Role of preoperative cessation of smoking and other factors in postoperative pulmonary complications: a blinded prospective study of coronary artery bypass patients. Mayo Clin Proc 1989;64:609–16.
[12] Burns DM. Cigarettes and cigarette smoking. Clin Chest Med 1991;12:631–42.
[13] Kaubam J. Effect of short term smoking halt on carboxyhemoglobin levels and P-50 values. Anesth Analg 1986;65:1186–8.
[14] Stein M, Cassara EL. Preoperative pulmonary evaluation and therapy for surgery patients. JAMA 1970; 211:787–90.
[15] Tarhan S, Moffitt EA, Sessler AD, et al. Risk of anesthesia and surgery in patients with chronic bronchitis and chronic obstructive pulmonary disease. Surgery 1973;74:720–6.
[16] Rojewski TE, Schuller DE, Clark RW, et al. Videoendoscopic determination of the mechanism of obstruction in obstructive sleep apnea. Otolaryngol Head Neck Surg 1984;92:127–31.
[17] Remmers JE, deGroot WJ, Sauerland EK, et al. Pathogenesis of upper airway occlusion during sleep. J Appl Physiol 1978;44:931–8.
[18] Li KK, Powell NB, Riley RW, et al. Overview of phase I surgery for obstructive sleep apnea syndrome. Ear Nose Throat J 1999;78:836–7, 841–5.
[19] Fairbanks DN. Uvulopalatopharyngoplasty complications and avoidance strategies. Otolaryngol Head Neck Surg 1990;102:239–45.
[20] Kirsch M, Guesnier L, LeBesnerais P, et al. Cardiac operations in octogenarians: perioperative risk factors for death and impaired autonomy. Ann Thorac Surg 1998;66:60–7.
[21] Weiss BM, Zemp L, Seifert B, et al. Outcome of pulmonary vascular disease in pregnancy: a systematic overview from 1978 through 1996. J Am Coll Cardiol 1998;31:1650–7.
[22] Krowka MJ, Plevak DJ, Findlay JY, et al. Pulmonary hemodynamics and perioperative cardiopulmonary-related mortality in patients with portopulmonary hypertension undergoing liver transplantation. Liver Transpl 2000;6:443–50.
[23] Goldman L, Caldera DL, Nussbaum SR, et al. Multifactorial index of cardiac risk in noncardiac surgical procedures. N Engl J Med 1977;297:845–50.
[24] Wong DH, Weber EC, Schell MJ, et al. Factors as-

[24] sociated with postoperative pulmonary complications in patients with severe chronic obstructive pulmonary disease. Anesth Analg 1995;80:276–84.
[25] Warner DO, Warner MA, Barnes RD, et al. Perioperative respiratory complications in patients with asthma. Anesthesiology 1996;85:460–7.
[26] Gerson MC, Hurst JM, Hertzberg VS, et al. Prediction of cardiac and pulmonary complications related to elective abdominal and noncardiac thoracic surgery in geriatric patients. Am J Med 1990;88:101–7.
[27] Djokovic JL, Hedley-Whyte J. Prediction of outcome of surgery and anesthesia in patients over 80. JAMA 1979;242:2301–6.
[28] Moulton MJ, Creswell LL, Mackey ME, et al. Obesity is not a risk factor for significant adverse outcomes after cardiac surgery. Circulation 1996; 94(9 Suppl):II87–92.
[29] Pasulka PS, Bistrian BR, Benotti PN, et al. The risks of surgery in obese patients. Ann Intern Med 1986; 104:540–6.
[30] Pooler HE. Relief of post-operative pain and its influence on vital capacity. BMJ 1949;2:1200–3.
[31] Wightman JA. A prospective survey of the incidence of postoperative pulmonary complications. Br J Surg 1968;55:85–91.
[32] Barone JE, Lincer RM. Correction: a prospective analysis of 1518 laparoscopic cholecystectomies. N Engl J Med 1991;325:1517–8.
[33] Phillips EH, Carroll BJ, Fallas MJ, et al. Comparison of laparoscopic cholecystectomy in obese and non-obese patients. Am Surg 1994;60:316–21.
[34] Brooks-Brunn JA. Predictors of postoperative pulmonary complications following abdominal surgery. Chest 1997;111:564–71.
[35] Berg H, Roed J, Viby-Mogensen J, et al. Residual neuromuscular block is a risk factor for postoperative pulmonary complications. A prospective, randomised, and blinded study of postoperative pulmonary complications after atracurium, vecuronium and pancuronium. Acta Anaesthesiol Scand 1997;41: 1095–103.
[36] Fisher BW, Majumdar SR, McAlister FA. Predicting pulmonary complications after nonthoracic surgery: a systematic review of blinded studies. Am J Med 2002;112:219–25.
[37] Bartlett RH, Gazzaniga AB, Geraghty TR. Respiratory maneuvers to prevent postoperative pulmonary complications. A critical review JAMA 1973;224: 1017–21.
[38] Bartlett RH, Morris AH, Fairley HB, et al. A prospective study of acute hypoxic respiratory failure. Chest 1986;89:684–9.
[39] Platell C, Hall JC. Atelectasis after abdominal surgery. J Am Coll Surg 1997;185:584–92.
[40] Pizov R, Takahashi M, Hirshman CA, et al. Halothane inhibition of ion transport of the tracheal epithelium. A possible mechanism for anesthetic-induced impairment of mucociliary clearance. Anesthesiology 1992;76:985–9.
[41] Gamsu G, Singer MM, Vincent HH, et al. Postoperative impairment of mucous transport in the lung. Am Rev Respir Dis 1976;114:673–9.
[42] Kotani N, Hashimoto H, Sessler DI, et al. Intraoperative modulation of alveolar macrophage function during isoflurane and propofol anesthesia. Anesthesiology 1998;89:1125–32.
[43] Eger 2nd EI. The pharmacology of isoflurane. Br J Anaesth 1984;56(Suppl 1):71S–99S.
[44] Knill RL. Control of breathing: effects of analgesic, anaesthetic and neuromuscular blocking drugs. Can J Anaesth 1988;35(3 [Pt 2]):S4–8.
[45] Knill RL, Kieraszewicz HT, Dodgson BG, et al. Chemical regulation of ventilation during isoflurane sedation and anaesthesia in humans. Can Anaesth Soc J 1983;30:607–14.
[46] Weil JV, McCullough RE, Kline JS, et al. Diminished ventilatory response to hypoxia and hypercapnia after morphine in normal man. N Engl J Med 1975;292: 1103–6.
[47] Giesecke Jr AH, Cale JO, Jenkins MT. The prostate, ventilation, and anesthesia. JAMA 1968;203:389–91.
[48] Pietak S, Weenig CS, Hickey R, et al. Anesthetic effects on ventilation in patients with chronic obstructive pulmonary disease. Anesthesiology 1975;42:160–6.
[49] Dueck R, Prutow RJ, Davies NJ, et al. The lung volume at which shunting occurs with inhalation anesthesia. Anesthesiology 1988;69:854–61.
[50] Hedenstierna G, Strandberg A, Brismar B, et al. Functional residual capacity, thoracoabdominal dimensions, and central blood volume during general anesthesia with muscle paralysis and mechanical ventilation. Anesthesiology 1985;62:247–54.
[51] Hedenstierna G. New aspects on atelectasis formation and gas exchange impairment during anaesthesia. Clin Physiol 1989;9:407–17.
[52] Brismar B, Hedenstierna G, Lundquist H, et al. Pulmonary densities during anesthesia with muscular relaxation–a proposal of atelectasis. Anesthesiology 1985;62:422–8.
[53] Strandberg A, Tokics L, Brismar B, et al. Atelectasis during anaesthesia and in the postoperative period. Acta Anaesthesiol Scand 1986;30:154–8.
[54] Krayer S, Rehder K, Vettermann J, et al. Position and motion of the human diaphragm during anesthesia-paralysis. Anesthesiology 1989;70:891–8.
[55] Tokics L, Hedenstierna G, Strandberg A, et al. Lung collapse and gas exchange during general anesthesia: effects of spontaneous breathing, muscle paralysis, and positive end-expiratory pressure. Anesthesiology 1987;66:157–67.
[56] Hedenstierna G, Tokics L, Strandberg A, et al. Correlation of gas exchange impairment to development of atelectasis during anaesthesia and muscle paralysis. Acta Anaesthesiol Scand 1986;30:183–91.
[57] Pien LC, Grammer LC, Patterson R. Minimal complications in a surgical population with severe asthma receiving prophylactic corticosteroids. J Allergy Clin Immunol 1988;82:696–700.

[58] Oh SH, Patterson R. Surgery in corticosteroid-dependent asthmatics. J Allergy Clin Immunol 1974; 53:345–51.

[59] Celli BR. Perioperative respiratory care of the patient undergoing upper abdominal surgery. Clin Chest Med 1993;14:253–61.

[60] Lubin M, Walker K, Smith R. Medical management of the surgical patient. Philadelphia: J. B. Lippincott; 1995.

[61] Xue FS, Li BW, Zhang GS, et al. The influence of surgical sites on early postoperative hypoxemia in adults undergoing elective surgery. Anesth Analg 1999;88:213–9.

[62] Rosenberg J, Ullstad T, Rasmussen J, et al. Time course of postoperative hypoxaemia. Eur J Surg 1994;160:137–43.

[63] Diaz O, Iglesia R, Ferrer M, et al. Effects of noninvasive ventilation on pulmonary gas exchange and hemodynamics during acute hypercapnic exacerbations of chronic obstructive pulmonary disease. Am J Respir Crit Care Med 1997;156:1840–5.

[64] Bergermann M, Donald PJ, aWengen DF. Screwdriver aspiration. A complication of dental implant placement. Int J Oral Maxillofac Surg 1992;21:339–41.

[65] Gillick MR. Rethinking the role of tube feeding in patients with advanced dementia. N Engl J Med 2000; 342:206–10.

[66] Orozco-Levi M, Torres A, Ferrer M, et al. Semirecumbent position protects from pulmonary aspiration but not completely from gastroesophageal reflux in mechanically ventilated patients. Am J Respir Crit Care Med 1995;152(4 Pt 1):1387–90.

[67] Mendelson C. The aspiration of stomach contents into the lungs during obstetric anesthesia. Am J Obstet Gynecol 1946;52:191–205.

[68] Doyle RL, Szaflarski N, Modin GW, et al. Identification of patients with acute lung injury. Predictors of mortality. Am J Respir Crit Care Med 1995; 152(6 Pt 1):1818–24.

[69] Bartlett JG. Anaerobic bacterial infections of the lung and pleural space. Clin Infect Dis 1993;16(Suppl 4): S248–55.

[70] Bowen TE, Fishback ME, Green DC. Treatment of refractory atelectasis. Ann Thorac Surg 1974;18:584–9.

[71] Wanner A, Landa JF, Nieman Jr RE, et al. Bedside bronchofiberscopy for atelectasis and lung abscess. JAMA 1973;224:1281–3.

[72] Jepsen S, Nielsen PH, Klaerke A, et al. [The effect of systemic N-acetylcysteine on postoperative expectoration. A prospective, randomized double-blind study]. [in Danish] Ugeskr Laeger 1989;151:1055–7.

[73] Jepsen S, Nielsen PH, Klaerke A, et al. Peroral N-acetylcysteine as prophylaxis against bronchopulmonary complications of pulmonary surgery. Scand J Thorac Cardiovasc Surg 1989;23:185–8.

[74] Kemper KJ, Ritz RH, Benson MS, et al. Helium-oxygen mixture in the treatment of postextubation stridor in pediatric trauma patients. Crit Care Med 1991;19:356–9.

[75] Rodeberg DA, Easter AJ, Washam MA, et al. Use of a helium-oxygen mixture in the treatment of postextubation stridor in pediatric patients with burns. J Burn Care Rehabil 1995;16:476–80.

[76] Timby J, Reed C, Zeilender S, et al. "Mechanical" causes of pulmonary edema. Chest 1990;98:973–9.

[77] McConkey PP. Postobstructive pulmonary oedema–a case series and review. Anaesth Intensive Care 2000;28:72–6.

[78] Willms D, Shure D. Pulmonary edema due to upper airway obstruction in adults. Chest 1988;94:1090–2.

[79] Holmes JR, Hensinger RN, Wojtys EW. Postoperative pulmonary edema in young, athletic adults. Am J Sports Med 1991;19:365–71.

[80] Wilson GW, Bircher NG. Acute pulmonary edema developing after laryngospasm: report of a case. J Oral Maxillofac Surg 1995;53:211–4.

[81] Cascade PN, Alexander GD, Mackie DS. Negative-pressure pulmonary edema after endotracheal intubation. Radiology 1993;186:671–5.

[82] Warner MA, Warner ME, Weber JG. Clinical significance of pulmonary aspiration during the perioperative period. Anesthesiology 1993;78:56–62.

[83] Ad Hoc Committee of the Scientific Assembly on Microbiology, Tuberculosis, and Pulmonary Infections. Hospital-acquired pneumonia in adults: diagnosis, assessment of severity, initial antimicrobial therapy, and preventive strategies. A consensus statement, American Thoracic Society, November 1995. Am J Respir Crit Care Med 1996;153:1711–25.

[84] Montravers P, Veber B, Auboyer C, et al. Diagnostic and therapeutic management of nosocomial pneumonia in surgical patients: results of the Eole study. Crit Care Med 2002;30:368–75.

[85] Carson JL, Kelley MA, Duff A, et al. The clinical course of pulmonary embolism. N Engl J Med 1992; 326:1240–5.

[86] Horlander KT, Mannino DM, Leeper KV. Pulmonary embolism mortality in the United States, 1979–1998: an analysis using multiple-cause mortality data. Arch Intern Med 2003;163:1711–7.

[87] Hirsh J, Dalen J, Anderson DR, et al. Oral anticoagulants: mechanism of action, clinical effectiveness, and optimal therapeutic range. Chest 2001; 119(1 Suppl):8S–21S.

[88] Hyers TM, Agnelli G, Hull RD, et al. Antithrombotic therapy for venous thromboembolic disease. Chest 2001;119(1 Suppl):176S–93S.

[89] Agnelli G, Prandoni P, Becattini C, et al. Extended oral anticoagulant therapy after a first episode of pulmonary embolism. Ann Intern Med 2003;139:19–25.

[90] Carr JB, Hansen ST. Fulminant fat embolism. Orthopedics 1990;13:258–61.

[91] Mellor A, Soni N. Fat embolism. Anaesthesia 2001; 56:145–54.

[92] Stojadinovic S, Hoer H, Eufinger H, et al. [Tracheobronchial perforations–a complication after mouth, maxillary and facial surgery]. [in German] Mund Kiefer Gesichtschir 1999;3:279–82.

[93] Massard G, Rouge C, Dabbagh A, et al. Tracheobronchial lacerations after intubation and tracheostomy. Ann Thorac Surg 1996;61:1483–7.

[94] Frick WG, Seals Jr RR. Smoking and wound healing: a review. Tex Dent J 1994;111:21–3.

[95] Moller AM, Pedersen T, Villebro N, et al. Effect of smoking on early complications after elective orthopaedic surgery. J Bone Joint Surg Br 2003;85:178–81.

[96] Delgado-Rodriguez M, Medina-Cuadros M, Martinez-Gallego G, et al. A prospective study of tobacco smoking as a predictor of complications in general surgery. Infect Control Hosp Epidemiol 2003;24:37–43.

[97] Moller AM, Maaloe R, Pedersen T. Postoperative intensive care admittance: the role of tobacco smoking. Acta Anaesthesiol Scand 2001;45:345–8.

[98] Warner MA, Divertie MB, Tinker JH. Preoperative cessation of smoking and pulmonary complications in coronary artery bypass patients. Anesthesiology 1984;60:380–3.

[99] Moller AM, Villebro N, Pedersen T, et al. Effect of preoperative smoking intervention on postoperative complications: a randomised clinical trial. Lancet 2002;359:114–7.

[100] Lancaster T. Individual behavioural counselling for smoking cessation. Cochrane Database Syst Rev 2002, Issue 3.

[101] Silagy C, Lancaster T, Stead L, et al. Nicotine replacement therapy for smoking cessation. Cochrane Database Syst Rev 2002, Issue 3.

[102] West R. Smoking cessation guidelines 2004 update. Edinburgh, Scotland: Health Scotland and ASH Scotland; 2004.

[103] Mendella LA, Manfreda J, Warren CP, et al. Steroid response in stable chronic obstructive pulmonary disease. Ann Intern Med 1982;96:17–21.

[104] Powell NB, Riley RW, Guilleminault C, et al. Obstructive sleep apnea, continuous positive airway pressure, and surgery. Otolaryngol Head Neck Surg 1988;99:362–9.

[105] Li KK, Riley RW, Powell NB, et al. Fiberoptic nasopharyngolaryngoscopy for airway monitoring after obstructive sleep apnea surgery. J Oral Maxillofac Surg 2000;58:1342–5 [discussion: 1345–6].

[106] Kearon C. Perioperative management of long-term anticoagulation. Semin Thromb Hemost 1998; 24(Suppl 1):77–83.

[107] Madura JA, Rookstool M, Wease G. The management of patients on chronic Coumadin therapy undergoing subsequent surgical procedures. Am Surg 1994;60:542–6 [discussion: 546–7].

[108] Celli BR, Rodriguez KS, Snider GL. A controlled trial of intermittent positive pressure breathing, incentive spirometry, and deep breathing exercises in preventing pulmonary complications after abdominal surgery. Am Rev Respir Dis 1984;130:12–5.

[109] Castillo R, Haas A. Chest physical therapy: comparative efficacy of preoperative and postoperative in the elderly. Arch Phys Med Rehabil 1985;66:376–9.

[110] Brooks-Brunn JA. Postoperative atelectasis and pneumonia. Heart Lung 1995;24:94–115.

[111] Aubier M, Viires N, Piquet J, et al. Effects of hypocalcemia on diaphragmatic strength generation. J Appl Physiol 1985;58:2054–61.

[112] Aubier M, Murciano D, Lecocguic Y, et al. Effect of hypophosphatemia on diaphragmatic contractility in patients with acute respiratory failure. N Engl J Med 1985;313:420–4.

[113] Pedersen T. Complications and death following anaesthesia. A prospective study with special reference to the influence of patient-, anaesthesia-, and surgery-related risk factors. Dan Med Bull 1994;41:319–31.

[114] Pedersen T, Eliasen K, Henriksen E. A prospective study of risk factors and cardiopulmonary complications associated with anaesthesia and surgery: risk indicators of cardiopulmonary morbidity. Acta Anaesthesiol Scand 1990;34:144–55.

[115] Hall JC, Tarala R, Harris J, et al. Incentive spirometry versus routine chest physiotherapy for prevention of pulmonary complications after abdominal surgery. Lancet 1991;337:953–6.

[116] Stock MC, Downs JB, Gauer PK, et al. Prevention of postoperative pulmonary complications with CPAP, incentive spirometry, and conservative therapy. Chest 1985;87:151–7.

[117] Cuschieri RJ, Morran CG, Howie JC, et al. Postoperative pain and pulmonary complications: comparison of three analgesic regimens. Br J Surg 1985;72: 495–8.

[118] Ballantyne JC, Carr DB, deFerranti S, et al. The comparative effects of postoperative analgesic therapies on pulmonary outcome: cumulative meta-analyses of randomized, controlled trials. Anesth Analg 1998;86: 598–612.

[119] Hirsh J. Prevention of venous thrombosis in patients undergoing major orthopaedic surgical procedures. Acta Chir Scand Suppl 1990;556:30–5.

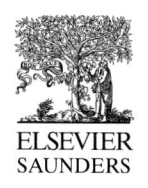

Prevention of Venous Thromboembolism

Divyang Sorathia, MD[a], Sujata Naik-Tolani, MD[b,c,*], Ramesh S. Gulrajani, MD[b,d]

[a]*Division of Pulmonary and Critical Care Medicine, The Brooklyn Hospital Center, Brooklyn, NY, USA*
[b]*Cornell University, New York, NY, USA*
[c]*Medical Intensive Care Unit, The Brooklyn Hospital Center, Brooklyn, NY, USA*
[d]*Department of Medicine, The Brooklyn Hospital Center, Brooklyn, NY, USA*

Venous thromboembolism (VTE) is a spectrum of disease that includes deep vein thrombosis (DVT) and pulmonary embolism (PE). To suspect DVT and not look for PE, or to suspect PE and not look for DVT, can lead to serious errors in patient management. VTE typically occurs in high-risk patients or in specific clinical situations. There is widespread agreement that patients who are at moderate or high risk for postoperative VTE should receive thromboprophylaxis while in the hospital [1]. Thromboprophylaxis in patients undergoing major surgery saves lives and reduces health care costs [2]. Preventing DVT, and thereby PE, in patients at risk clearly is preferable to treating the condition after it has appeared [3], a view supported by cost-effectiveness analysis [3–6]. It is suggested that in the present day and age, failure to provide appropriate thromboprophylaxis is negligence [7].

To discuss VTE prophylaxis in its entirety is beyond the scope of this article. Discussion, therefore, is limited to those clinical situations that are applicable to oral and maxillofacial surgery patients.

Pathogenesis and natural history of venous thromboembolism

Venous stasis begins in the vicinity of a venous valve or at the site of intimal injury, leading to platelet aggregation and the release of chemical mediators, such as interleukin 1 and tumor necrosis factor. The coagulation cascade is activated and a thrombus forms. Three scenarios can occur: a small thrombus may be swept into the pulmonary vasculature, resulting in an asymptomatic PE; complete obstruction of the vessel may occur; or partial obstruction of the vessel may occur with growth of the thrombus. The thrombus (all or part of it) can embolize at any time during this period; the highest risk is during the first 72 hours. Once a reasonable size, the thrombus undergoes fibrinolytic resolution or organization with recanalization and re-endothelialization. Anticoagulation therapy halts thrombus growth allowing fibrinolysis to occur unopposed. The extent of the residual venous obstruction determines the risk for recurrent DVT.

Epidemiology

A first time VTE occurs in approximately 100 persons per 100,000 each year in the United States [8]. It is estimated that as many as 600,000 episodes of PE occur annually in the United States, resulting in

* Corresponding author. Division of Pulmonary and Critical Care Medicine, The Brooklyn Hospital Center, 121 Dekalb Avenue, Brooklyn, NY 11201.
E-mail address: sun9003@nyp.org (S. Naik-Tolani).

100,000 to 200,000 deaths [9]. Of patients who have first-time VTE, 26% to 47% have idiopathic VTE [8].

The prevalence of asymptomatic DVT on admission to the hospital is high in elderly patients, especially those over, age 80 and very low in patients under age 55 [10]. The incidence rates of DVT increase exponentially with age, from less than five cases annually per 100,000 in persons less than 15 years of age to nearly 450 to 600 cases annually per 100,000 in persons 80 years of age [11,12]. There seems to be no significant difference in the incidence of VTE in men and women [8].

Hirst and colleagues report a higher prevalence of PE in North Americans (15%) than in Japanese (0.7%) [13]. There is a low incidence of VTE in Hispanic and Asian and Pacific Islander populations (compared with white and African American populations). This is not understood fully but may relate to genetic factors predisposing to VTE, such as factor V Leiden, which occurs in 0.5% of the Asian population versus 5% of the white population [14–16].

There are varying reports regarding the effect of seasons on the incidence of VTE. Some studies [17,18] note a higher incidence of fatal PE in the winter months; however, Bounamaeux and coworkers do not observe any seasonal variation in the incidence of VTE [19]. Possible explanations for a higher incidence of VTE in the winter months include venous stasis resulting from decreased physical activity, vasoconstriction induced by the cold weather, and hypercoagulability triggered by respiratory tract infections [20].

Despite anticoagulation therapy, VTE recurs frequently in the first few months after the initial event, with a recurrence rate of nearly 7% at 6 months [8].

Mortalities related to VTE are attributed mostly to missed diagnosis rather than to inadequate treatment [21]. Death occurs within 1 month of diagnosis in nearly 6% of DVT cases and 12% of PE cases [8]. Early mortality after VTE is associated strongly with PE as the initial presentation, advanced age, malignancy, and underlying cardiovascular disease [8].

In the absence of prophylaxis, the incidence of hospital-acquired DVT is approximately 10% to 40% in medical or general surgery and 40% to 60% after major orthopedic surgery [1,11].

Incidence of venous thromboembolism in oral and maxillofacial surgery patients

The incidence of DVT and PE in major oral and maxillofacial surgery is low [22]. In 1995, the British reported 60 cases of PE in 79% of 130 maxillofacial surgical units over a 5-year period. Of these 60 cases, 58.3% had undergone surgery for malignancy, 25% followed trauma, and 6.7% had undergone orthognathic surgery. In two patients (3.3%), PE followed parotid surgery. Of the remaining four patients, one had a bone-grafting procedure at the time of closure of an oronasal fistula, another had a skin graft from an unspecified site for sulcoplasty, and one was unspecified. One case followed third molar excision in which no major risk factors were highlighted. Of the 103 units, 64% reported no cases of DVT in the patients during the 5 years and 68% reported no instances of PE. This study estimates the incidence of VTE, as a complication associated with all oral and maxillofacial surgical procedures under general anesthesia, to be in the range of 0.00035% to 0.06% at worst [22].

Risk factors for venous thromboembolism

In 1856, Rudolf Virchow proposed the risk triad that predisposes to VTE: (1) venous stasis, (2) endothelial injury, and (3) hypercoagulability.

In 1990, the landmark study, Prospective Investigation of Pulmonary Embolism Diagnosis (PIOPED), identified the most common risk factors for VTE as immobilization, surgery within the past 3 months, stroke, history of prior VTE, and malignancy [23]. The Nurses' Health study notes three additional risk factors for VTE—obesity, cigarette smoking, and hypertension [24]. Hospital or nursing home confinement, surgery, trauma, malignant neoplasm, chemotherapy, neurologic disease with paresis, central venous catheter or pacemaker, varicose veins, and superficial vein thrombosis are independent and important risk factors for VTE [25].

The components of Virchow's triad (single or combined) are the underlying mechanisms of the risk factors known today (Fig. 1).

Risk factors that seem to result from venous stasis include age greater than 40 years, immobility, cardiac or respiratory failure, and varicose veins. It is suggested that a combination of decreased mobility and muscle tone with increase in morbidity and degenerative vascular changes is responsible for the age-related increase in the incidence of VTE [26]. Autopsy studies note a prevalence of VTE ranging from 15% to 80% in those patients confined to bed for long periods of time [27,28]. Cardiac and respiratory failures are controversial risk factors for VTE. After controlling for hospitalization, congestive heart failure or other cardiac diseases are not found to

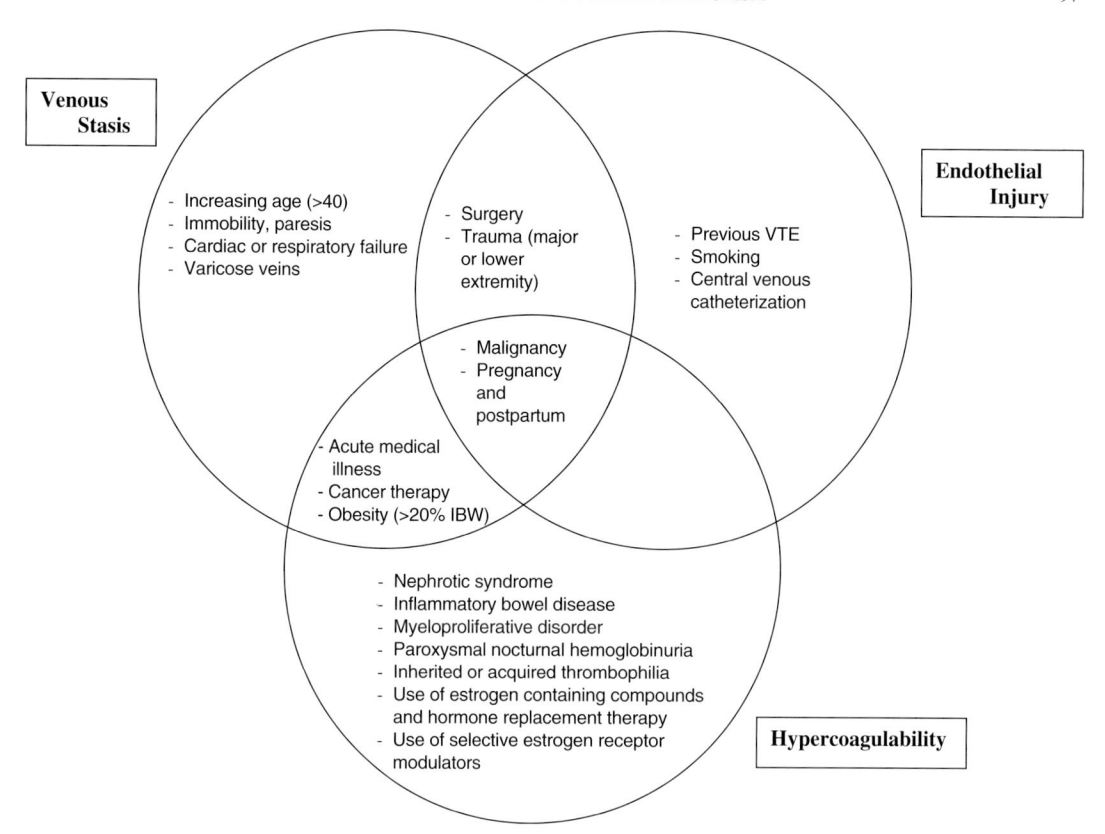

Fig. 1. Risk factors for venous thromboembolism according to Virchow's risk triad. (*Data from* Geerts WH, Pineo GF, Heit JA, et al. Prevention of venous thromboembolism. The Seventh ACCP Conference on Antithrombotic and Thrombolytic Therapy Chest 2004;126:338–400S; and Michota FA. Venous thromboembolism prophylaxis in the medically ill patient. Clin Chest Med 2003;24:93–101.)

be an independent risk factor for VTE [25,29]. In contrast, autopsy studies demonstrate an increased prevalence of PE in patients who have cardiac disease [30,31].

Surgery and trauma result in endothelial injury and venous stasis. With cancer, malignancy and surgery are likely to be the strongest risk factor for VTE. The risk for thrombosis is not limited to the immediate postoperative period but continues for several weeks [32]. Studies show that nearly 60% of subjects who have major trauma have DVT of the lower extremities, which, in most cases, is asymptomatic [33]. The factors associated with an increased risk for VTE in patients who have trauma are increasing age, surgery, blood transfusion, fracture of the femur and tibia, and spinal cord injury [33].

Central venous catheterization, a history of previous VTE, and smoking are responsible for endothelial injury. Since the 1970s, there has been an increased recognition of upper extremity DVT [34–38]. The increased incidence is attributed to the use of central venous catheters and transvenous pacemakers [34]. The risk for PE associated with upper limb venous thrombosis is estimated at between 9% and 36% [39–42]. One study shows that the risk for thrombosis is higher with femoral vein catheters (21%) than with subclavian vein catheters (1.9%) [43]. Venous thrombosis is the most common complication of Hickman catheter used in patients who have solid tumors [44]. A prior VTE is an independent risk factor for further thrombotic events [11,45,46].

An alteration in the coagulation cascade resulting in a hypercoagulable state is seen in nephrotic syndrome, inflammatory bowel disease, myeloproliferative disorders, paroxysmal nocturnal hemoglobinuria, thrombophilia, the use of estrogen-containing compounds, hormone replacement therapy, and selective estrogen receptor modulators. Evaluation for thrombophilic conditions should be limited to those patients who have recurrent VTE or a strong family history of VTE [47].

Hypercoagulable state and venous stasis seem to be the underlying mechanisms for acute medical illness, cancer therapy, and obesity as risk factors for VTE. A weight of greater than 20% of ideal body weight predisposes individuals to VTE. There is emerging biologic and clinical data that suggests an association between obstructive sleep apnea and VTE [48].

All three components of the triad contribute to malignancy, pregnancy, and the postpartum period in their risk for VTE. Although thrombosis occurs most commonly in the setting of advanced malignant disease, it also may be the first sign of an underlying cancer that may predate the diagnosis by several years [49]. An evaluation for occult malignancy is warranted for patients presenting with recurrent idiopathic VTE [49–53].

Risk factors for VTE during pregnancy include advanced maternal age, high parity, obesity, operative delivery, history of prior VTE, and thrombophilia [54]. The incidence of VTE is threefold to eightfold higher in the postpartum period compared with the antepartum period [55].

Risk factors for venous thromboembolism in oral and maxillofacial surgery patients

Many procedures in oral and maxillofacial surgery of a relatively minor nature are performed in young adults who rapidly mobilize postoperatively and, therefore, have few risk factors for the development of VTE. Advances in maxillofacial surgery, however, have led to longer operations on older patients who are less resilient and mobilize more slowly and have multiple operative sites, including the pelvis (simple bone grafts and vascularized composite free flaps), lower limb (grafts from metatarsals, tibia, and fibula), and abdomen (jejunal transfer, rectus abdominis myocutaneous, and full-thickness skin grafts). These are major risk factors in the etiology and pathogenesis of VTE [22].

Risk factor stratification

Patients may have one or more risk factors for VTE, and these factors are cumulative. Patients can be risk stratified into groups based on patient age, type of hospital service that is providing care for the primary surgical or medical disorder, type of surgery, and presence of additional risk factors [56]. Patients can be risk stratified as follows.

Low risk

- Minor surgery in patients younger than 40 years old who have no additional risk factors

Moderate risk

- Minor surgery in patients 40 to 60 years old or who have additional risk factors
- Major surgery in patients younger than 40 years old who have no additional risk factors
- Any neurosurgical patients who have less than 2 additional risk factors
- Any patients who have medical illness, are critically ill, or have burns with one additional risk factor
- Patients who have trauma without additional risk factors

High risk

- Minor surgery in patients older than 60 years of age
- Major surgery in patients older than 40 years or who have additional risk factors
- Patients who have malignancy
- Any patients who have medical illness, are critically ill, have burns, or have undergone neurosurgery who have two or more additional risk factors
- Trauma patients who have one or more additional risk factors

Highest risk

- Surgery in patients who have multiple risk factors
- Patients who have lower extremity, pelvic trauma, or major head injury

Prevention of venous thromboembolism

Primary prophylaxis is the implementation of various strategies to prevent DVT. It is preferred in most clinical situations and is more cost effective than treatment of VTE.

Secondary prophylaxis involves the early detection and treatment of subclinical venous thrombosis and the prevention of the embolic and postphlebitic sequel.

Prophylaxis methods

An ideal method for VTE prophylaxis is one that can be administered easily to maximize compliance by physicians, patients, and nurses. The method should be safe and without the need for laboratory monitoring. Finally, it should be the most cost effective compared with other methods.

Surveillance is clinical vigilance and aggressive investigation for patients who have signs and symptoms suspicious of VTE. Routine screening for DVT by Duplex ultrasonography of the lower extremities is not recommended as a part of routine prophylaxis [56]. Early and persistent mobilization should be an integral part of the care of all patients who have risk factors for VTE. Teamwork is needed to mobilize patients as soon as possible. There are only a few randomized trials that show that early mobilization and physical therapy reduce the risk for VTE.

Mechanical methods

Mechanical methods for prophylaxis enhance the outflow within the lower extremities venous system to reduce the stasis in the veins. Mechanical methods include graduated compression stockings (GCS), intermittent pneumatic compression (IPC) devices, and venous foot pump. Leg IPC stimulates fibrinolytic activity, which is related to a reduction in plasminogen activator inhibitor-1 levels associated with a resulting increase in tissue plasminogen activator activity [57]. Thus, leg IPC has local and systemic effects. Mechanical methods for prophylaxis are shown to reduce the risk for DVT [1,58–65]. They are less efficacious, however, than the anticoagulation-based option for the prevention of DVT [1,63, 66–68].

Bleeding as a side effect is not a concern with these devices and, therefore, they are the thromboprophylaxis of choice for patients who have bleeding or are at high risk for bleeding. Mechanical methods also are recommended as an adjunct to anticoagulant-based prophylaxis [56].

The proper use of these devices includes choosing the correct size, appropriate application, removal for a short interval every day, and ensuring that the use of these devices does not prevent early mobilization. GCS should be used with caution in patients who have arterial insufficiency [69–71]. Mechanical devices are contraindicated if patients have been on bed rest or immobilized for more than 72 hours without any form of prophylaxis, because it may cause a newly formed clot to dislodge. In such situations, the authors recommend lower extremity Duplex ultrasonography before the application of a mechanical device.

Vena cava interruption

Interruption of the inferior vena cava (IVC) to prevent PE arising from DVT was proposed in 1868 [72]. Today, several different kinds of vena cava filters are available in the United States, including retrievable filters.

Currently, indications for IVC filter (IVCF) placement in patients who have documented VTE include absolute contraindication to anticoagulation, life-threatening hemorrhage on anticoagulation, or recurrent VTE despite therapeutic anticoagulation.

IVC interruption does not prevent further DVT formation and does not prevent thromboembolization from sources proximal to the device. Many investigators recommend continuing anticoagulation, if not contraindicated, after IVCF placement; however, this is controversial [73]. The long-term safety and efficacy of IVCFs remain uncertain; their use should be restricted to situations in which anticoagulation clearly is contraindicated [73] or has failed to control VTE.

Many patients have only temporary contraindications to anticoagulation. In these situations, it is wise to insert a temporary (retrievable) IVCF. It can be left in place for up to 6 weeks [74]. Studies demonstrate them to be safe and effective [75].

Prophylactic IVCF insertion is recommended by some for use in trauma patients who are at very high risk for VTE. McMurtry and colleagues, however, find no difference in the rates of PE in patients who do or do not have IVCFs; and an increased risk for thrombosis at the insertion site is noted with the use of IVCFs [76]. IVCFs are not recommended for primary prophylaxis in surgical or trauma patients [56].

Pharmacologic agents

Aspirin and other antiplatelet drugs

Aspirin and other antiplatelet drugs are highly effective at reducing major vascular events in patients who are at risk for or who have established atherosclerotic disease [77]. The inferior efficacy of aspirin compared with other methods for VTE prophylaxis is demonstrated in clinical trials [78,79]. The use of aspirin alone as a prophylaxis is not recommended [56].

Antithrombotic agents

There are many antithrombotic agents available for the prevention of VTE, with important differences in efficacy and in the frequency of their principle side effect—bleeding. Antithrombotic agents, such as low molecular weight heparin (LMWH), fondaparinux, and direct thrombin inhibitors, are cleared primarily by the kidney.

Dosing of antithrombotic agents. For each of the antithrombotic agents, clinicians should consider the manufacturer's suggested dosing guidelines. In patients who have renal impairment, the doses of LMWH, fondaparinux, direct thrombin inhibitors, and other antithrombotic drugs that are cleared by the kidneys need to be adjusted. This is true particularly in elderly patients and those who are at high risk for bleeding [56].

Heparins. Unfractionated heparin (UFH) is a heterogenous mixture of polysaccharide chains. For decades, 5000 U of UFH administered subcutaneously every 8 to 12 hours has been a standard and well accepted mode of VTE prophylaxis in a wide range of surgical procedures [80]. Such prophylaxis is effective in patients who are at low to moderate risk for VTE. A reduction in incidence of DVT form 22% to 9% is demonstrated [80].

LMWHs are fractionated natural heparin created by depolymerization. They have a superior bioavailability, with a rapid onset of action and longer half-life allowing a convenient once-daily dosing.

Monitoring of activated partial thromboplastin time (PTT) is not necessary with either UFH or LMWH. In 1995, Warkentin and coworkers demonstrated a lower incidence of heparin-induced thrombocytopenia in patients taking LMWH versus UFH [81]. Most studies demonstrate no significant difference in the incidence of major bleeding with the use of LMWH versus UFH [82,83].

Vitamin K antagonist. Warfarin is the single most commonly used vitamin K antagonist (VKA) for the treatment and prophylaxis of VTE. It has a slow onset of action, interacts with many foods and drugs, and requires monitoring of coagulation profile and dose adjustment. As a method of prophylaxis against VTE, warfarin is used in the group of patients who are at highest risk for VTE. To be effective, a target INR of 2.5 (INR range, 2.0 to 3.0) must be maintained.

Direct thrombin inhibitors. Direct thrombin inhibitors are a group of anticoagulants that seem to be more active than heparin. Currently, four Food and Drug Administration (FDA)-approved direct thrombin inhibitors are available (argatroban, lepirudin, bivalirudin, and desirudin). Desirudin is found to be safe and superior to UFH [84,85] and more effective than enoxaparin in prevention of DVT after total hip replacement [86].

Ximelagartan is an orally administered direct thrombin inhibitor. It seems to be effective for VTE prevention after orthopedic surgery. It was rejected by the FDA in 2004, however, because of the concerns of about hepatotoxicity.

Factor Xa inhibitors. Currently, the only commercially available member of this class is fondaparinux, which is a synthetic pentasaccharide that inhibits activated factor X. It is administered subcutaneously and has a long half-life of approximately 17 hours, allowing for once-daily dosing. This drug is approved by the FDA only for VTE prophylaxis in total hip or knee arthroplasty and hip fracture surgery. It has not been adopted widely because of concerns about high bleeding rates, lack of an antidote, cost, risks associated with neuraxial anesthesia, and delayed clearance in patients who have renal impairment [87].

Danaparoid is a low molecular weight heparinoid that is not available commercially in the United States. It is shown in animal studies to be more effective than heparins in preventing the extension of experimentally induced venous thrombosis [88].

Rationale for thromboprophylaxis

As discussed previously, DVT occurs commonly in hospitalized patients. Risk factors and clinical situations that predispose to VTE are now well known. The morbidity, mortality, and costs that are incurred as a result of DVT and its complications are high. Screening tools do not prevent VTE and fatal PE can occur without any warning. Treatment for thromboembolic diseases is not free of complications. Fortunately, today, highly efficacious and cost-effective methods for prophylaxis are available. Appropriately used thromboprophylaxis has a high risk-benefit ratio. In that PE is the most common preventable cause of hospital death, it is only appropriate that thromboprophylaxis is routine for patients at risk for VTE.

Recommended prophylaxis in various clinical situations

Weighing the degree of risk for VTE versus the different methods for VTE prophylaxis and their potential adverse effects, it is critical to match the

Table 1
Recommended venous thromboembolism prophylaxis in various clinical situations

Clinical situations	Recommended prophylaxis
Low risk	
Minor surgery in patients <40 years who have no ARF	Early and persistent mobilization
Moderate risk	
Minor surgery in patients 40–60 years or who have ARF or	LDUH 5000 U bid or LMWH ≤3400 U once daily
Major surgery in patients <40 years who have no ARF or	
Any patient who has medical illness, is critically ill, or has burns with one ARF	
Any neurosurgic patient who has less than two ARF	IPC with or without GCS
High risk	
Minor surgery in patients >60 years or	LDUH 5000 U tid or LMWH >3400 U daily
Major surgery in patients >40 years or ARF or	
Patients who have malignancy or	
Any patient who has medical illness, is critically ill, or has burns with two or more ARF	
Any neurosurgical patient who has two or more ARF	IPC or GCS with LDUH or LMWH
Trauma patients who have one or more ARF[a]	LMWH as soon as it is safe, until discharge/IPC or GCS
Highest risk	
Surgery in patients who have multiple risk factors[b]	LDUH 5000 U tid or LMWH >3400 U daily with IPC or GCS
Patients who have lower extremity, pelvic trauma, or major head injury[c]	LMWH/IPC or GCS/screening for DVT/no IVCF/post discharge prescription

Abbreviations: ARF, additional risk factors; LDUH, low dose unfractionated heparin.
[a] Use of IPC or GSC if LMWH prophylaxis is delayed or contraindicated.
[b] Selected high-risk patients (major cancer surgery) need post discharge prophylaxis with LMWH.
[c] IVCFs as primary prophylaxis is not recommended; postdischarge prophylaxis with LMWH or VKA (target INR 2.5, INR range 2.0–3.0).
Data from Geerts WH, Pineo GF, Heit JA, et al. Prevention of Venous Thromboembolism. The Seventh ACCP Conference on Antithrombotic and Thrombolytic Therapy. Chest 2004;126:338S–400S.

intensity of thromboprophylaxis with the degree of risk for venous thrombosis, keeping in mind the risk-benefit ratio.

Table 1 outlines the recommendations for prevention of VTE in various clinical situations. In the event that a recommended anticoagulant-based prophylaxis cannot be instituted because of contraindications, patients should receive mechanical methods for prophylaxis, even though they are less efficacious.

For patients who have malignancy, hip fracture, or trauma and for those in the postpartum period, there are some additional recommendations.

Malignancy

Patients who have malignancy often have long-term indwelling central venous catheters. Even though theses catheters are an independent risk factor for VTE, the routine use of prophylaxis is not recommended [56].

Hip fracture surgery

Hip fracture surgery patients are at very high risk for VTE. Prophylaxis for VTE should be initiated at time of admission to the hospital even if surgery is likely to be delayed. Fondaparinux, high-dose LMWH, or VKA is the recommended agent [56].

Trauma

Trauma patients who are at high risk for VTE and have not received optimal prophylaxis since the trauma may have asymptomatic DVT. It is recommended that this group of patients undergo screening Duplex ultrasonography [56].

Pregnancy

As discussed previously, patients in the postpartum period are at higher risk for VTE than during

Table 2
Recommended venous thromboembolism prophylaxis during pregnancy

Clinical situations	Recommended prophylaxis
I. History of prior venous thromboembolism	
Single episode of VTE associated with a transient risk factor	Surveillance + PPA
If previous episode was pregnancy or estrogen related or there are additional risk factors	Prophylactic LMWH
Single idiopathic episode of VTE, not on long-term anticoagulants or Single episode of VTE in women who have thrombophilia or a strong family history of thrombophilia, not on long-term anticoagulants	Prophylactic LMWH + PPA
Antithrombin-deficient women	Prophylactic LMWH
Multiple episodes of VTE or on long-term anticoagulants	Adjusted dose UFH or LMWH + PPA
II. No history of prior venous thromboembolism	
Antithrombin-deficient women	Prophylactic LMWH
Presence of thrombophilia	Surveillance or prophylactic LMWH + PPA

All women should use graduated elastic stockings.
Terminology: adjusted dose LMWH, weight-adjusted, full-treatment dose, enoxaparin 1 mg/kg SC, q 12 hourly; adjusted dose UFH, UFH SC q 12 hourly in doses adjusted to target a midinterval aPTT into the therapeutic range; postpartum anticoagulation (PPA), warfarin for 4 to 6 weeks with a target INR of 2.5 (range 2.0 to 3.0) with initial UFH or LMWH overlap until INR is ≥2.0; prophylactic LMWH, enoxaparin 40 mg SC q 24 hourly; surveillance, clinical vigilance and aggressive investigation of women with symptoms suspicious of VTE.
Data from Bates SM, Greer IA, Hirsch J, Ginsberg JS. Use of antithrombotic agents during pregnancy. The Seventh ACCP Conference on Antithrombotic and Thrombolytic Therapy. Chest 2004;126:627S–44S.

the antepartum period. Table 2 outlines the guidelines for VTE prophylaxis during pregnancy.

Duration of prophylaxis

In a surgical setting, prophylaxis ideally is started before surgery and continued until patients are completely ambulatory [1]. Trauma patients often require inpatient rehabilitation before discharge or may even have impaired mobility after discharge. In these patients, it is recommended that prophylaxis is continued during these periods with either LMWH or VKA [56]. Patients undergoing hip fracture surgery should receive prophylaxis for up to 28 to 35 days after surgery with fondaparinux, LMWH, or VKA [56]. In surgical patients who have malignancy, prophylaxis with LMWH for 2 to 3 weeks after hospital discharge seems to reduce the incidence of asymptomatic DVT [56].

Strategies to improve venous thromboembolism prophylaxis in hospitals

Appropriate implementation of VTE prophylaxis in hospital settings is a major concern. Tooher and colleagues reviewed strategies to improve the practice of VTE prophylaxis from 1996 to May 2003. They conclude that the passive dissemination of guidelines is unlikely to improve VTE prophylaxis practice. Several active strategies used together, which incorporate some method of reminding clinicians to assess patients for DVT risk and assisting the selection of appropriate prophylaxis, are likely to result in the achievement of optimal outcomes [89]. Geerts and colleagues recommend that all hospitals develop a formal strategy, in the form of a written policy, that addresses the prevention of VTE. A strategy of this kind also is likely to protect caregivers and hospitals from legal liability [56]. The authors recommend the use of preprinted order sheets or computerized admission orders that include VTE prophylaxis.

Summary

VTE is a preventable cause of in-hospital morbidity and mortality. Even though the incidence of VTE in oral and maxillofacial surgery patients is low, most patients have identifiable risk factors, such as malignancy and trauma. Using the appropriate preventive methods (degree of risk matched to the intensity of prophylaxis, high risk-benefit ratio) the incidence of VTE and the postphlebitic syndrome can be reduced. A formal strategy (written policy, preprinted order form, or computerized admission orders) that addresses the issue is the key to successful implementation of VTE prophylaxis.

References

[1] Geerts WH, Heit JA, Clagett GP, et al. Prevention of venous thromboembolism. Chest 2001;119:132S–75S.

[2] Bergqvist D, Jendteg S, Lindgren B, et al. The economics of general thromboembolic prophylaxis. World J Surg 1988;12:349–55.

[3] Salzman EW, Davies GC. Prophylaxis of venous thromboembolism: analysis of cost effectiveness. Ann Surg 1980;191:207–18.

[4] Hull RD, Hirsch J, Sackett DL, et al. Cost effectiveness of primary and secondary prevention of fatal pulmonary embolism in high-risk surgical patient. Can Med Assoc J 1982;127:990–5.

[5] Bergqvist D, Matzsch T, Jendteg S, et al. The cost effectiveness of prevention of post-operative thromboembolism. Acta Chir Scand 1990;556(Suppl):36–41.

[6] Paiement GD, Wessinger SJ, Harris WH. Cost effectiveness of prophylaxis in total hip replacement. Am J Surg 1991;161:519–24.

[7] Parker Williams J, Vickers R. Major orthopaedic surgery on the leg and thromboembolism. BMJ 1991;303: 531–2.

[8] White RH. The epidemiology of venous thromboembolism. Circulation 2003;107:I-4–I-8.

[9] Fedullo PF, Tapson VF. The evaluation of suspected pulmonary embolism. N Engl J Med 2003;349:1247–56.

[10] Oger E, Bressollette L, Nonent M, et al. High prevalence of asymptomatic deep vein thrombosis on admission in a medical unit among elderly patients. Thromb Haemost 2002;88:592–7.

[11] Anderson FA, Wheeler HB, Goldberg RJ, et al. A population-based perspective of the hospital incidence and case-fatality rates of deep vein thrombosis and pulmonary embolism: the Worcester DVT Study. Arch Intern Med 1991;151:933–8.

[12] Silverstein MD, Hiet JA, Mohr DN, et al. Trends in the incidence of deep vein thrombosis and pulmonary embolism: a 25 year population-based study. Arch Intern Med 1998;158:585–93.

[13] Hirst AE, Gore I, Tanaka K, et al. Myocardial infarction and pulmonary embolism. Arch Pathol 1965;80:365–70.

[14] Ridker PM, Miletich JP, Hennekens CH, et al. Ethnic distribution of Factor V Leiden in 4047 men and women. Implication for venous thromboembolism screening. JAMA 1997;277:1305–7.

[15] Gregg JP, Yamane AJ, Grody WW. Prevalence of the factor V Leiden mutation in four distinct Am ethnic population. Am J Med Genet 1997;73:334–6.

[16] Angchaisuksiri P, Pingsuthiwong S, Aryuchai K, et al. Prevalence of the G1691A mutation in the factor V gene (factor V Leiden) and the G20210A prothrombin gene mutation in the Thai population. Am J Hematol 2000;65:119–22.

[17] Wroblewski BM, Siney P, White R. Seasonal variation in fatal pulmonary embolism after hip arthroplasty. Lancet 1990;335:56.

[18] Gallerani M, Manfredini R, Ricci L, et al. Sudden death from pulmonary thromboembolism: chronobiological aspects. Eur Heart J 1992;13:661–5.

[19] Bounameaux H, Hicklin L, Desmarais S. Seasonal variation in deep vein thrombosis. BMJ 1996;312:284–5.

[20] Boulay F, Berthier F, Schoukroun G, et al. Seasonal variations in hospital admission for deep vein thrombosis and pulmonary embolism: analysis of discharge data. BMJ 2001;323:601–2.

[21] Carson JL, Kelley MA, Duff A, et al. The clinical course of pulmonary embolism: one year follow-up of PIOPED patients. N Engl Med 1992;326:1240–5.

[22] Lowry JC. Thromboembolic disease and thromboprophylaxis in oral and maxillofacial surgery: experience and practice. Br J Oral Maxillofac Surg 1995;33: 101–6.

[23] The PIOPED Investigators. Value of the ventilation/perfusion scan in acute pulmonary embolism. Results of the prospective investigation of pulmonary embolism diagnosis (PIOPED). JAMA 1990;263:2753–9.

[24] Goldhaber SZ, Grodstein F, Stampfer MJ, et al. A prospective study of risk factors for pulmonary embolism in women. JAMA 1997;277:642–5.

[25] Heit JA, Silverstein MD, Mohr DN, et al. Risk factors for deep vein thrombosis and pulmonary embolism. Arch Intern Med 2000;160:809–15.

[26] Rosendaal FR. Venous thrombosis: a multicausal disease. Lancet 1999;353:1167–73.

[27] Gibbs NM. Venous thrombosis of the lower limbs with particular reference to bed rest. Br J Surg 1957; 45:209.

[28] Sevitt S. Thrombosis and embolism after injury. J Clin Pathol 1970;4:86–101.

[29] Grady D, Wenger NK, Herrington D, et al. Postmenopausal hormone therapy increases the risk for venous thromboembolic disease. Ann Intern Med 2000;132: 689–96.

[30] Coon WW. Risk factors in pulmonary embolism. Surg Gynecol Obstet 1976;143:385–90.

[31] Coon WW, Coller FA. Some epidemiologic considerations of thromboembolism. Surg Gynecol Obstet 1959;109:487–501.

[32] Bergqvist D, Benoni G, Bjorgell O, et al. Low-molecular weight heparin (enoxaparin) as prophylaxis against venous thromboembolism after total hip replacement. N Engl J Med 1996;335:696–700.

[33] Geerts WH, Code KI, Jay RM, et al. A prospective study of venous thromboembolism after major trauma. N Engl J Med 1994;331:1601–6.

[34] Campbell CB, Chandler JG, Tegtemyer CJ, et al. Axillary, subclavian, and bracheocephalic vein obstruction. Surgery 1997;82:816–26.

[35] Kroger K, Schelo C, Rudofsky G. Colour Doppler sonographic diagnosis of upper limb venous thrombosis. Clin Sci (Lond) 1998;94:657–61.

[36] Huber P, Hauptli W, Schmitt HE, et al. Die Axillar-Subclaviavenenthrombose und ihre Folgen. Internist (Berl) 1987;28:336–43.

[37] Theis SW, Zaus M, Kiefhaber M, et al. Primare und sekundare Schultergurtelvenenthrombose: eine

Analyse von 227 patienten. [abstract]. Vasa 1994; 43(Suppl):102.

[38] Layher T, Heinrich F. Retrspektive Betrachtung von Armbzw-Schultervenenthrombosen am Krankenhaus Bruchasal im Zeitraum von 1973 und 1993 [abstract]. Vasa 1994;43(Suppl):103.

[39] Prandoni P, Polistena P, Bernardi E, et al. Upper extremity deep vein thrombosis: risk factors, diagnosis, and complications. Arch Intern Med 1997;157:57–62.

[40] Becker DM, Philbrick JT, Walker FB. Axillary and subclavian venous thrombosis: prognosis and treatment. Arch Intern Med 1991;151:1934–43.

[41] Monreal M, Lafoz E, Ruiz J, et al. Upper-extremity deep venous thrombosis and pulmonary embolism: a prospective study. Chest 1991;99:280–3.

[42] Horattas MC, Wright DJ, Fenton AH, et al. Changing concepts of deep vein thrombosis of the upper extremity: report of a series and review of the literature. Surgery 1988;104:561–7.

[43] Merre J, De Jonghe B, Golliot F, et al. Complications of femoral and subclavian venous catheterization in critically ill patients: a randomized controlled trial. JAMA 2001;286:700–7.

[44] Anderson AJ, Krasnow SH, Boyer MW, et al. Thrombosis: the major Hickman catheter complication in patients with solid tumor. Chest 1989;95:71–5.

[45] Hull RD, Raskob GE, Gent M, et al. Effectiveness of intermittent pneumatic leg compression for preventing deep vein thrombosis after total hip replacement. JAMA 1990;263:2313–7.

[46] Nicolaides AN, Irving D. Clinical factors and the risk of deep venous thrombosis. In: Nicolaides AN, editor. Thromboembolims: aetiology, advances in prevention and management. Lancaster: MTP Press; 1975.

[47] Wuhl J, Graham MG. Pulmonary embolism: new diagnostic tools and treatment paradigms. Resid Staff Physician 2005;51:14–21.

[48] Caples SM, Kara T, Somers VK. Cardiopulmonary consequences of obstructive sleep apnea. Am J Respir Crit Care Med (seminars) 2005;26:25–32.

[49] Prandoni P, Lensing AWA, Buller HR, et al. Deep-vein thrombosis and the incidence of subsequent symptomatic cancer. N Engl J Med 1992;327:1128–33.

[50] Nordstrom M, Lindblad B, Anderson H, et al. Deep venous thrombosis and occult malignancy: an epidemiological study. BMJ 1994;308:891–4.

[51] Sorensen HT, Mellemkjaer L, Steffensen FH, et al. The risk of a diagnosis of cancer after primary deep venous thormbosis or pulmonary embolism. N Engl J Med 1998;338:1169–73.

[52] Hettiarachchi RJ, Lok J, Prins MH, et al. Undiagnosed malignancy in patients with deep vein thrombsis: incidence, risk indicators, and diagnosis. Cancer 1998;83:180–5.

[53] Schulman S, Lindmarker P. Incidence of cancer after prophylaxis with warfarin against recurrent venous thromboembolism: Duration of Anticoagulation Trial. N Engl J Med 2000;342:1953–8.

[54] Kujovich JL. Hormones and pregnancy: thromboembolic risks for women. Br J Haematol 2004;126: 443–54.

[55] McColl MD, Ramsay JE, Tait RC, et al. Risk factors for pregnancy associated venous thromboembolism. Thromb Haemost 1997;78:1183–8.

[56] Geerts WH, Pineo GF, Heit JA, et al. Prevention of venous thromboembolism. The Seventh ACCP Conference on Antithrombotic and Thrombolytic Therapy. Chest 2004;126:338S–400S.

[57] Comerota AJ, Chouhan V, Harada RN, et al. The fibrinolytic effects of intermittent pneumatic compression: mechanism of enhanced fibrinolysis. Ann Surg 1997;226:306–14.

[58] Coe NP, Collins RE, Klein LA, et al. Prevention of deep vein thrombosis in urological patients: a controlled, randomized trial of low-dose heparin and external pneumatic compression boots. Surgery 1978;83:230–4.

[59] Turpie AG, Hirsh J, Gent M, et al. Prevention of deep vein thrombosis in potential neurosurgical patients: a randomized trial comparing graduated compression stockings alone or graduated compression stockings plus intermittent pneumatic compression with control. Arch Intern Med 1989;149:679–81.

[60] Vanek VW. Meta-analysis of effectiveness of intermittent pneumatic compression devices with a comparison of thigh-high to knee-high sleeves. Am Surg 1998;64:1050–8.

[61] Warwick D, Harrison J, Glew D, et al. Comparison of the use of a foot pump with the use of low-molecular-weight heparin for the prevention of deep-vein thrombosis after total hip replacement. J Bone Joint Surg Am 1998;80:1158–66.

[62] Agu O, Hamilton G, Baker D. Graduated compression stockings in the prevention of venous thromboembolism. Br J Surg 1999;86:992–1004.

[63] Freedman KB, Brookenthal KR, Fitzgerald RH, et al. A meta-analysis of thromboembolic prophylaxis following elective total hip arthroplasty. J Bone Joint Surg Am 2000;82:929–38.

[64] Westrich GH, Haas SB, Mosca P, et al. Meta-analyses of thromboembolic prophylaxis after total knee arthroplasty. J Bone Joint Surg Br 2000;82:795–800.

[65] Amarigiri SV, Lees TA. Elastic compression stockings for prevention of deep vein thrombosis. Cochrane Database Syst Rev 2001 (1) [Database online].

[66] Hull RD, Raskob GE, Gent M, et al. Effectiveness of intermittent pneumatic leg compression for preventing deep vein thrombosis after total hip replacement. JAMA 1990;263:2313–7.

[67] Blanchard J, Meuwly JY, Leyvraz PF, et al. Prevention of deep-vein thrombosis after total knee replacement. Randomised comparison between a low-molecular-weight heparin (nadroparin) and mechanical prophylaxis with a foot-pump system. J Bone Joint Surg Br 1999;81:654–9.

[68] Iorio A, Agnelli G. Low-molecular-weight and unfractionated heparin for prevention of venous thromboembolism in neurosurgery: a meta-analysis. Arch Intern Med 2000;160:2327–32.

[69] Kay TW, Martin FI. Heel ulcers in patients with longstanding diabetes who wear antiembolism stockings. Med J Aust 1986;145:290–1.

[70] Heath DI, Kent SJ, Johns DL, et al. Arterial thrombosis associated with graduated pressure antiembolic stockings. BMJ 1987;295:580.

[71] Merrett ND, Hanel KC. Ischaemic complications of graduated compression stockings in the treatment of deep venous thrombosis. Postgrad Med J 1993;69:232–4.

[72] Trousseau A. In: Phlegmatia alba dolens: clinique medicale de l'Hotel-Dieu de Paris. Paris: J.B. Baillere et Fils; 1868. p. 652–95.

[73] Streiff MB. Vena caval filters: a comprehensive review. Blood 2000;95:3669–77.

[74] Millward SF. Temporary and retrievable inferior vena cava filters: current status. J Vasc Interv Radiol 1998; 9:381–7.

[75] Bovyn G, Gory P, Reynaud P, et al. The Tempofilter: a multicenter study of a new temporary caval filter implantable for up to six weeks. Ann Vasc Surg 1997;11: 520–8.

[76] McMurtry AL, Owings JT, Anderson JT, et al. Increased use of prophylactic vena cava filters in trauma patients failed to decrease overall incidence of pulmonary embolism. J Am Coll Surg 1999;189:314–20.

[77] Patrono C, Coller B, Dalen JE, et al. Platelet-active drugs: the relationships among dose, effectiveness, and side effects. Chest 2001;119(Suppl):39S–63S.

[78] Graor RA, Stewart JH, Lotke PA, et al. RD heparin (ardeparin sodium) vs aspirin to prevent deep venous thrombosis after hip or knee replacement surgery [abstract]. Chest 1992;102:118S.

[79] Gent M, Hirsh J, Ginsberg JS, et al. Low-molecular weight heparinoid orgaran is more effective than aspirin in the prevention of venous thromboembolism after surgery for hip fracture. Circulation 1996;93:80–4.

[80] Collins R, Scrimgeour A, Yusuf S, et al. Reduction in fatal pulmonary embolism and venous thrombosis by perioperative administration of subcutaneous heparin: overview of results of randomized trials in general, orthopedic, and urologic surgery. N Engl J Med 1988; 318:1162–73.

[81] Warkentin TE, Levine MN, Hirsh J, et al. Heparin induced thrombocytopenia in patients treated with low-molecular weight heparin or unfractionated heparin. N Engl J Med 1995;332:1330–5.

[82] Nurmohamed MT, Rosendaal FR, Buller HR, et al. Low-molecular-weight heparin versus standard heparin in general and orthopedic surgery: a meta-analysis. Lancet 1992;340:152–6.

[83] Kakkar VV, Cohen AT, Edmonson RA, et al. Low molecular weight versus standard heparin for prevention of venous thromboembolism after major abdominal surgery. Lancet 1993;341:259–65.

[84] Eriksson BI, Ekman S, Kalebo P, et al. Prevention of deep vein thrombosis after total hip replacement: direct thrombin inhibition with recombinant hirudin, CGP 39393. Lancet 1996;347:635–9.

[85] Eriksson BI, Ekman S, Lindbratt S, et al. Prevention of thromboembolism with use of recombinant hirudin. Results of a double-blind, multi-center trial comparing the efficacy of desirudin (Revasc) with that of unfractionated heparin in patients having a total hip replacement. J Bone Joint Surg Am 1997;79:326–33.

[86] Eriksson BI, Wille-Jorgensen P, Kalebo P, et al. A comparision of recombinant hirudin with a low-molecular weight heparin to prevent thromboembolic complications after total hip replacement. N Engl J Med 1997;337:1329–35.

[87] Kaboli PJ, Brenner A, Dunn AS. Prevention of venous thromboembolism in medical and surgical patients. Cleve Clin J Med 2005;72(1):S7–13.

[88] Boneu B, Buchanan MR, Cade JF, et al. Effects of heparin, its low molecular weight fractions and other glycosaminoglycans on thrombus growth in vivo. Thromb Res 1985;40:81–9.

[89] Tooher R, Middleton P, Pham C, et al. A systematic review of strategies to improve prophylaxis for venous thromboembolism in hospitals. Ann Surg 2005;241: 397–415.

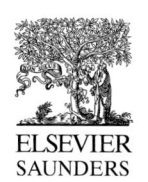

Wound Healing and Perioperative Care

Vivek Shetty, DDS, DrMedDent[a],*, Harry C. Schwartz, DMD, MD, FACS[a,b]

[a]*University of California, Los Angeles, CA, USA*
[b]*Southern California Permanente Medical Group, Los Angeles, CA, USA*

Wounding or injury unleashes a tightly choreographed array of cellular, physiologic, biochemical, and molecular processes directed toward restoring the integrity and functional capacity of the damaged tissue. Healing in the orofacial region usually is taken for granted, yet a variety of local and systemic factors can hinder the process of tissue restitution and set the stage for adverse outcomes. Although surgical attention invariably focuses on local wound care, consideration of systemic factors is equally important. An understanding of the biologic underpinnings of the wound-healing continuum provides surgeons with a framework for developing the skills required to care for wounds and facilitate healing.

How do wounds heal?

Wound healing starts immediately after injury and generally progresses in an established sequence of overlapping phases: hemostasis, inflammation, proliferation, and remodeling. Kane's analogy of wound healing to the repair of a damaged house provides a simple framework for understanding the complex interplay of the cellular events that comprise healing (Table 1) [1].

As with a house destroyed by a natural disaster, the initial response is directed toward minimizing further damage by capping off the broken vascular conduits. Functioning as utility workers, arriving platelets go about sealing off the damaged blood vessels. They secrete substances to augment the reflexive vasoconstriction of the injured vessels and aggregate rapidly at the wound site, adhering to each other and the exposed vascular subendothelial collagen to form a primary platelet plug organized within a fibrin matrix. The clot secures hemostasis and provides a provisional matrix through which succeeding reparative cells can migrate. Degranulating platelets initiate the subsequent reparative steps by releasing various cytokines and growth factors, including interleukins, transforming growth factor-beta (TGF-β), and platelet-derived growth factor. Unless there are underlying clotting disorders, hemostasis usually is complete within minutes of the initial injury.

Once hemostatis is secured, the inflammatory phase begins and lasts for up to 4 days post injury. Clinically, the inflammatory phase is characterized by pain, heat, redness, and swelling. Cytokines released at the wound site sequentially recruit neutrophils and monocytes to the site of injury. Arriving neutrophils or polymorphonucleocytes serve as the nonskilled laborers involved in site preparation. They swarm around the site and clean up the rubble. Aided by local mast cells, the neutrophils ingest tissue debris and microorganisms by phagocytosis and provide the first line of defense against infection. As they perish, the short-lived neutrophils release proinflamatory cytokines that continue to stimulate the inflammatory response. Around this time, the general contractor cell or macrophage is established at the site and begins to direct the subsequent activities of the specialized subcontractor cells. The macrophages, essentially activated monocytes, continue with the wound microdébridement initiated by the neutrophils. In ad-

* Corresponding author. 23-009 UCLA School of Dentistry, 10833 Le Conte Avenue, Los Angeles, CA 90095-1668.
 E-mail address: vshetty@ucla.edu (V. Shetty).

Table 1
Kane's analogy of wound-healing phases to house restoration

Healing phase	Time	Principal cells	House-building analogy
Hemostasis	Immediate	Platelets	Capping of damaged conduits
Inflammation	Day 1–4	Neutrophils	Unskilled laborers for site cleanup
Proliferation/ granulation	Day 4–22	Macrophages Lymphocytes	Supervisor Specific site preparation
		Angiocytes	Plumbers
		Neurocytes	Electricians
		Fibroblasts	Framers
		Keratinocytes	Roofers
Remodeling	Day 22– 2 years	Fibrocytes	Remodelers

Adapted from: Kane D. Chronic wound healing and chronic wound management. In: Krasner D, Rodeheaver GT, Sibbald RG, editors. Chronic wound care: a clinical source for healthcare professionals. 3rd edit. Wayne (PA): Health Management Publications; 2001. p. 7–17.

dition, they release a slew of growth factors and cytokines (TGF-β, fibroblast growth factor, interleukin 1, insulin-like growth factor I and II, and so forth) that stimulate and direct the succeeding proliferative phase [2].

Beginning as early as the third day post injury and lasting up to 3 weeks, the proliferative phase is distinguished by the formation of pink, granular tissues containing inflammatory cells, fibroblasts, and budding vasculature enclosed in a loose matrix. Using a housing-building analogy, the framer cells or fibroblasts move into the cleared site and, working under the direction of the general contractor, begin the framing or reinforcing of the wound with collagen fibers. Concomitantly, specialized cells, such as the angiocytes and neurocytes, install new plumbing and wiring through the framework. As the framing proceeds, the epidermal cells begin their task as roofers and help provide a protective outside barrier through re-epithelialization.

Once the basic infrastructure of the wound is established, the wound enters the remodeling phase and most activity moves inwards. Through progressive remodeling and strengthening of the framework, the immature scar tissue eventually is replaced by a more refined and organized tissue that is closer to the native tissue. The fibroblasts are the principal facilitators of the remodeling phase, which can last for several years. They act as the source of collagen and the proteoglycans that make up the extracellular matrix. Homeostasis of scar collagen and extracellular matrix is regulated to a large extent by serine proteases and matrix metalloproteinases under the control of regulatory cytokines. Tissue inhibitors of the matrix metalloproteinases provide a tight control of proteolytic activity within the scar. Any disruption of this orderly balance can lead to excess or inadequate matrix degradation and can result in either an exuberant scar or wound dehiscence.

Factors associated with impaired healing can be grouped into two classes, local and systemic. Local factors include the presence of foreign bodies, tissue maceration, wound ischemia, and increased bioburden. Systemic factors include advanced age, malnutrition, and coexisting diseases. Good surgical practice involves a proactive assessment of the impact of these cofactors on healing and, when possible, making use of clinical strategies to remove or reduce the impact of these factors.

What interferes with wound healing?

Wound bioburden

All bacteria impose a metabolic load on wounds because they compete with new tissue for nutrients and oxygen and produce byproducts that are harmful to the normal physiologic balance of the healing wound. The bacterial burden, also known as wound bioburden [3], provokes various degrees of inflammation in the wounded tissue through released endotoxins and metalloproteinases that can degrade fibrin and local wound growth factors. The fibrin matrix is essential for fibroblast migration and macrophage phagocytic activity. Newly formed cells and their collagen matrix, in particular, are susceptible to these breakdown products of wound infection. Depending on local tissue conditions and the quality of the host immune response, the wound bioburden can progress from a simple contamination to critical colonization and, eventually, frank infection. The clinical diagnosis of wound infection usually is made on the basis of the presenting signs (induration, pus, pain, and erythema) and can be confirmed by a wound culture that shows greater than 10^5 organisms per gram of tissue [4,5].

All wounds, in particular oral wounds, are contaminated, and the progression to frank infection in a contaminated wound can be visualized as a set of scales. The beneficial effects of local wound care and host immunocompetence tip the scale in the direction of healing. Alternatively, the quantity and mix of the infecting microorganisms and infection-potentiating factors, such as hematoma, necrotic tissue, and foreign bodies, tilt the balance toward infection. Other local factors that may allow the wound-infection continuum to advance after oral surgery include continued tissue trauma from prostheses, avascular bone chips in fractures or osteotomies, and implanted biomaterials. Some bioimplants irritate wounds mechanically, whereas others solubilize in the biologic environment and provoke a chemical irritation. Even biocompatible devices, such as bone plate and screws, can act as a nidus for infection. Once an implant-associated infection develops, it is difficult to control without removal of the foreign body. To the extent possible, all elective incisions should be placed to avoid trauma under function.

A competent immune system and antibiotics are no substitute for meticulous surgical technique and proper wound toilet. To minimize the effects of the wound bioburden, the treatment should be based on sound surgical principles. Techniques include careful wound débridement, diluting the bacterial counts by copious wound irrigation before closure, and systemic antibiotics used, when necessary, in tandem with local antiseptics. If antibiotics are administered, they must be given before surgery or shortly after the injury, because adequate tissue levels of the antibiotic are not achieved for up to 90 minutes after an intravenous dose [6].

Age

As people age, the entire healing process occurs more slowly. The major components of the healing response in aging skin or mucosa are deficient or damaged with progressive injuries [7]. As a result, free oxidative radicals continue to accumulate and are harmful to the dermal enzymes responsible for the integrity of the dermal or mucosal composition. In addition, the regional vascular support may be subjected to extrinsic deterioration and systemic disease decompensation, resulting in poor perfusion capability [8]. Beyond the gradual decline in the physiologic processes, elderly patients have a greater incidence of chronic conditions, including cardiovascular disease, pulmonary disease, and diabetes. The systemic disease frequently compounds the deterioration in the regional vascular support and the restricted tissue perfusion can impair healing. In elderly patients undergoing maxillofacial surgery, preemptive steps to prevent complicated healing include minimizing, where possible, extensive stripping of the periosteal and soft tissue envelope [9].

Poor tissue perfusion and oxygenation

Oxygen plays a critical role in all phases of the wound-healing cascade—inflammation, fibroplasia, epithelialization, angiogenesis, and remodeling [10,11]. Poor oxygenation interferes with the synthesis of collagen because oxygen is required for the hydroxylation of lysine and proline [12]. Wounds in hypoxic tissues are infected more easily and heal poorly as leukocytic, fibroblastic, and epithelial proliferation is depressed by low oxygen concentration. Delayed movement of neutrophils, opsonins, and the other mediators of inflammation to the wound site further diminishes the effectiveness of the phagocytic defense system and allows bacteria to proliferate. Most healing problems associated with diabetes mellitus, irradiation, small vessel atherosclerosis, chronic infection, and cardiovascular disease can be attributed to local tissue ischemia.

The local microcirculation after injury influences the wound's ability to resist the inevitable bacterial proliferation. Tissue traumatized by rough handling, or desiccated by cautery or prolonged air drying, tends to be poorly perfused and susceptible to infection. Similarly, tissue ischemia can be produced by tight or improperly placed sutures and poorly designed flaps. Hypovolemia, anemia, and peripheral vascular disease all affect wound healing adversely. Especially in trauma patients, therapy must be focused on keeping the wounds perfused with oxygenated blood. Cold, pain, and fear all induce catecholamine release, leading to increased sympathetic tone and increasing the peripheral vasoconstriction and tissue hypoxia. Peripheral blood flow can be improved by keeping patients warm and controlling pain and anxiety. It is important to maintain patients' cardiac output and intravascular volume. Anemia per se is not a cofactor in impaired healing; however, severe anemia (<20 mg/dL) should be corrected by transfusion. Patients evidencing clinical hypovolemia require fluid replacement therapy, because the depleted intravascular volume reduces the transport oxygen and nutrients to the tissues and has an impact on the cellular activities needed for healing.

Smoking tobacco is another common contributor to decreased tissue oxygenation [13]. After every cigarette, the peripheral vasoconstriction can last up to 1 hour; thus, a pack-a-day smoker remains tissue hypoxic for most of each day. Cigarette smoke contains carbon monoxide, which binds to hemoglobin, reducing the oxygen-carrying capacity of the blood.

Whenever possible, smokers should be asked to abstain from smoking for a minimum of 1 week before and after surgical procedures.

Concomitant disease

Wound healing can be impaired by a variety of systemic conditions, including diabetes mellitus, peripheral vascular disease, and immune compromise. Diabetics are predisposed to atherosclerosis and microangiopathy, which are associated with tissue hypoxia. There is impaired wound healing and an increased rate of wound infection in diabetics. The tissue hyperglycemia in poorly controlled diabetes affects the immune system adversely, including neutrophil and lymphocyte function, and increases the risk of infection [14]. Uncontrolled blood glucose hinders red blood cell permeability and impairs blood flow through the critical small vessels at the wound surface. The hemoglobin release of oxygen is impaired, resulting in an oxygen and nutrient deficit in the healing wound. The wound ischemia and impaired recruitment of cells resulting from the small vessel occlusive disease renders the wound vulnerable to bacterial and fungal infections. Well-controlled diabetics have a far lower incidence of wound-healing problems. Improving diabetic control before elective surgery reduces the incidence of wound-healing problems, although it does not reverse the microangiopathy.

Similarly, patients who have chronic renal failure and uremia have a disrupted immune response as manifested by depressed neutrophil function, leucopenia related to complement activation, diminished T and B lymphocyte function, and a reduction in natural killer cell activity. The attenuation of the inflammatory response makes these patients more susceptible to infection [15].

Patients who have a debilitated immune system include those who have HIV or AIDS and are in advanced stages of the disease, those on immunosuppressive therapy, those who have cancer or chronic disease, and those taking high-dose steroids for extended periods [16]. Immunocompromised patients are unable to mount an adequate immune response and all phases of healing are delayed. Studies indicate that HIV-infected patients who have CD4 counts less than 50 cells/μL are at significant risk of poor wound outcome [17].

Poor nutrition

Various nutrients are required for different phases of the healing process. Nutritional deficiencies severe enough to lower serum albumin to less than 2 g/dL are associated with a prolonged inflammatory phase, decreased fibroplasia, impaired neovascularization, collagen synthesis, and wound remodeling. In malnourished patients, protein is diverted from cellular repair to providing the glucose required for cellular maintenance, further compounding the healing process. Lack of vitamin A depresses the inflammatory response, whereas the B-complex vitamins and cobalt are essential cofactors in antibody formation, white blood cell function, and bacterial resistance. Inadequate vitamin C can cause a lysis of collagen, such that fresh wounds have delayed collagen formation and healed wounds can break down. Trace minerals, including copper, iron, and manganese, are required as cofactors for producing enzymes necessary for all phases of wound healing. Data suggests that zinc repletion, in states of deficiency, returns healing to its normal rate [18]. Alternatively, exceeding the zinc levels can exert a distinctly detrimental effect on healing by inhibiting macrophage migration and interference with collagen cross-linking.

If possible, elective surgery should be postponed until nutritional deficiencies are corrected. Even a few days of repletion ameliorates wound-healing problems in malnourished patients [19]. Postoperatively, it is important to resume enteral feeding as soon as possible. If there are difficulties with swallowing or oropharyngeal wounds, a feeding tube can be useful. Total parenteral nutrition may be necessary if the gastrointestinal system must be bypassed.

Radiation injury

The effects of therapeutic radiation are permanent and related directly to the dose [20]. Impaired surgical wound healing can be seen at total doses above 5000 cGy. There is damage to the small blood vessels of the dermis and submucosa, with obliterative endarteritis and a decrease in overall vascular supply. The epithelium becomes thinned and fragile. Radiated tissues are traumatized easily, producing ulcers that are slow to heal. The dermis and submucosa become thickened and fibrotic with damaged fibroblasts [21]. Hypoxic, fibrotic tissue is less able to support normal wound healing and is predisposed to infection.

Hence, surgeons always must anticipate the possibility of a complicated healing after surgery or traumatic injury in irradiated tissue. Wound dehiscence is common and wounds heals slowly or incompletely. Even minor trauma may result in ulceration and colonization by opportunistic bacteria. If patients cannot mount an effective inflammatory response, progressive necrosis of the tissues may follow. Healing can be achieved only by excising all nonvital tissue and covering the bed with a well-vascularized flap. Because of the relative hypoxia at the irradiated site, tissue with intact blood supply may need to be brought in to provide oxygen and the cells necessary for inflammation and healing.

Medications

Many drugs can impair the wound-healing process and, when possible, should be discontinued before elective surgery. Nonsteroidal anti-inflammatory drugs and other platelet inhibitors affect hemostasis and predispose to hematoma formation. They are best stopped 1 week before surgery. Depending on a patient's international normalized ratio, coumadin usually is stopped 2 or 3 days before surgery and substituted by low molecular weight heparin until hours before surgery. Anticoagulants are resumed as soon as the risk of surgical bleeding is over. Although a short course of perioperative steroids (used to reduce intracranial pressure or decrease surgical edema) has minimal effect on wound healing, chronic steroids inhibit almost every phase of wound healing and increase the risk of infection. Steroids suppress the inflammatory response, reduce immunocompetent lymphocytes, and decrease fibroplasia, collagen formation, and neovascularity [22]. Fibroblasts reach the site in a delayed fashion, and wound strength is decreased by as much as 30%. Epithelialization and wound contraction also are impaired. Unfortunately, chronic steroids rarely can be discontinued for surgery.

Antineoplastic agents exert their cytotoxic effect by interfering with the cell cycle. The reduction in protein synthesis or cell division manifests as impaired proliferation of fibroblasts and collagen formation in the healing wound. Attendant neutropenia also predisposes to wound infection by prolonging the inflammatory phase of wound healing. Chemotherapy also affects wound healing indirectly when nausea and vomiting produce malnutrition. Fortunately, the effects of these agents on wound healing are confined to the treatment period and immediately thereafter. Elective surgery often can be scheduled between cycles of therapy.

Intravenous bisphosphonates, zoledronic acid and pamidronate disodium, are used to prevent pathologic fracture in patients who have multiple myeloma or tumor metastases to bone. Their antiangiogenic properties and their capacity to abrogate the normal bone remodeling can produce recalcitrant osteonecrosis of the jaws. Affected patients should not have incisions in the tissues overlying the jawbones. Although there is no direct effect on wound healing, exposed bone becomes necrotic and wounds in the overlying tissues fail to close. Stopping the drug for as long as 6 months does not seem to reverse the pathologic process.

Principles of wound care

Most simple wounds, such as surgical incisions or clean lacerations, heal rapidly by primary intention. Complex wounds, such as burns, avulsions, and infected or contaminated injuries, may heal more slowly by secondary intention and may require skin grafts or flaps before they can heal. Current wound management focuses on three principles: control or elimination of causative factors, systemic support to reduce existing cofactors, and maintaining a physiologic local wound environment. An increased understanding of the wound-healing processes, however, has led to greater interest in manipulating the wound microenvironment to facilitate healing. Traditional passive ways of treating wounds rapidly are giving way to approaches that enhance healing beyond its normal maximal inherent rate through the use of growth factors, extracellular matrix components, living skin equivalents, and bioabsorbable collagen scaffolds.

Wound closure

The basic principles of wound closure are important particularly in the head and neck, where the goal is a mechanically sound wound closure and a cosmetically acceptable scar. All wounds should be rendered clean as possible, débriding them of nonviable tissue or foreign bodies. In some instances, wet-to-dry dressings are preferable to surgical débridement. Copious saline irrigation should be used to dilute bacterial and other particulate contaminants. Ragged wound margins must be revised. Undermining of wound margins may be required to achieve a tension-free closure. With revised wound margins and undermining, the dermal (subcutaneous) sutures should approximate the wound. All dead space should be eliminated. Depending on the nature of the wound, sutures, suction drains, or pressure dressings may be used for this purpose.

Where appropriate, closure of wounds should be performed in a layered manner. Deep sutures are placed best in strong, fibrous tissue: fascia or dermis rather than muscle or fat. Wound tensile strength depends on suture integrity in the first few weeks, until new collagen is remodeled sufficiently. Hence, polyglycolic acid sutures work well for this purpose. Nonresorbable sutures may be indicated in cases where a wound is under tension. Catgut is obsolete for most deep wound closures because it resorbs rapidly. Closure of the dermal (subcutaneous) layer is the key to esthetic wound closure. Dermal sutures should be inverted to avoid extrusion of the knots. Depending on the skin thickness, they are not necessarily placed as close as possible to the surface. Sutures that are too close to the surface can become extruded or cause a stitch abscess. These sutures should be placed in the vascular, collagenous dermis and should reach no higher than the lowest level of the epidermis. Maintaining the deeper portion of these sutures wider than the superficial portion encourages eversion and approximation of the epidermis. Wound margins needing revision should be beveled slightly away from the surface to help evert and approximate the epidermis. A mismatch in suturing this level is noted easily in the subsequent scar and should be avoided if esthetics are important. Inversion of wound margins delays wound healing and produces a wider scar.

Esthetic closure of the epidermal layer can be achieved in many ways. With proper dermal closure, skin sutures (and their cross-hatches) can be avoided in favor of porous tape. A running subcuticular suture can be placed. Skin sutures can be placed for 1 or 2 days and then replaced by tape. Fast resorbing catgut sutures can be placed. When the type and location of a wound calls for a strong epithelial closure, there are other options. Mucosa can be closed with either permanent or resorbable sutures. Skin can be closed with permanent sutures or staples. If the deeper portion of the suture is wider than the portion that crosses the surface, there is slight eversion of the wound margins. The design of skin staples also fosters wound eversion. Depending on an individual wound, simple sutures, horizontal or vertical mattress sutures, half-buried mattress sutures, or running sutures can be used.

Partial-thickness wounds

Partial-thickness injuries include those caused by abrasions and by the harvesting of skin or mucosal grafts. Such injuries heal by epithelialization from wound margins and from epidermal appendages, such as hair follicles, ducts, and pores in the wound bed. After hemostasis, partial-thickness wounds of the skin form a scab. Epithelialization takes place beneath the scab. In the moist environment of the mucosa, similar wounds form a fibrinous pseudomembrane. Dressings may be useful in making partial-thickness wounds more comfortable and in aiding epithelialization. Gauze dressings impregnated with various antibacterial substances and occlusive plastic films often are used for this purpose. The risk of dressings is that bacteria can proliferate beneath them; hence, dressings should be used with care to avoid infection. Wet-to-dry dressings are effective in débriding partial-thickness wounds that become infected. The bacterial count in a wound should be reduced below 10^5 per gram. Healing then can proceed normally. Systemic antibiotics do not work well for this and should be used only if there is cellulitis in the surrounding tissues [23].

Full-thickness wounds

Full-thickness injuries imply a complete loss of the epithelium and its appendages. Subcutaneous (submucosal) tissues, fat, fascia, muscle, bone, cartilage, organs, and other tissues may be exposed in the wound bed. Full-thickness wounds can be caused by tumor resection, trauma, burns, infection, radiation, or vascular compromise. Left alone, these injuries heal gradually by granulation and epithelialization. This process is slow and can be uncomfortable. Infection may intervene before the protective epithelium is restored. Full-thickness wounds heal more rapidly if they are covered by epithelium. If the wound bed is clean and well vascularized, a full- or partial-thickness skin graft can be placed. Depending on the location, a flap that carries its own blood supply could be a better choice. As with split-thickness wounds, the bacterial count in infected or contaminated wounds must be reduced below 10^5 per gram before they can be closed. Systemic antibiotics do not lower these bacterial counts significantly; dressing changes and topical antibacterial agents are more useful.

Scars

Scarring is an inevitable consequence of healing. The strength and appearance of scars differ, depending on the location and type of injury and the presence of intrinsic and extrinsic factors in the host. If wound healing is problematic or takes place under excessive tension, the esthetics of the scar is affected. Such scars tend to be thick, wide, raised, and a poor color match with the surrounding tissues.

Every region of the body has relaxed skin tension lines. The placement of elective incisions parallel to these lines improves the appearance of the ultimate scar. In the case of traumatic wounds or of incisions that cross these lines, the appearance of the ultimate scar is worse. Z-plasty or other techniques that reorient the wound can be useful in improving the appearance of the scar.

Keloids are scars that grow beyond the boundaries of the original wound, bulging above and invading the surrounding tissue. Keloids are caused by uncontrolled deposition of collagen (that is not balanced by collagen lysis) in an otherwise healed wound. Africans and dark-skinned people especially are prone to forming keloids. A variety of intralesional and topical steroids, antihistamines, pressure, surgical excision, and radiation all are used to treat this condition with varying degrees of success. Scars that are thickened so that they bulge above the level of the surrounding tissue are called hypertrophic scars. In contrast to keloids, hypertrophic scars do not extend beyond the boundaries of the original wound and they soften and flatten over time. Hypertrophic scars respond to treatment far better than keloids. Surgical reorientation within the relaxed skin tension lines and intralesional steroids are effective in managing hypertrophic scarring.

References

[1] Kane D. Chronic wound healing and chronic wound management. In: Krasner D, Rodeheaver GT, Sibbald RG, editors. Chronic wound care: a clinical source for healthcare professionals. 3rd edition. Wayne (PA): Health Management Publications; 2001. p. 7–17.

[2] Werner S, Grose R. Regulation of wound healing by growth factors and cytokines. Physiol Rev 2003;83: 835–70.

[3] Browne A, Dow G, Sibbald R. Infected wounds: definitions and controversies. In: Falanga V, editor. Cutaneous wound healing. London: Martin Dunitz; 2001. p. 203–19.

[4] Robson MC, Krizek TK, Heggers JP. Biology of surgical infection. In: Ravitch MM, editor. Current problems in surgery. Chicago: Yearbook Medical Publishers; 1973. p. 1–62.

[5] Bowler PG. The 105 bacterial growth guideline: reassessing its clinical relevance in wound healing. Ostomy Wound Manage 2003;49:44–53.

[6] Ehrlich HP, Licko V, Hunt TK. Kinetics of cephaloradine in experimental wounds. Am J Med Sci 1975; 265:33–44.

[7] Reed MJ, Koike T, Puolakkainen P. Wound repair in aging. A review. Methods Mol Med 2003;78:217–37.

[8] Fenske NA, Lober CW. Structural and functional changes of normal aging skin. J Am Acad Dermatol 1986;15(4 Pt 1):571–85.

[9] Bradley JC. Age changes in the vascular supply of the mandible. Br J Oral Surg 1972;12:142–4.

[10] Hunt TK, Conolly WB, Aronson SB, et al. Anaerobic metabolism and wound healing: a hypothesis for the initiation and cessation of collagen synthesis in wounds. Am J Surg 1978;135:328–32.

[11] Gottrup F. Oxygen, wound healing and the development of infection. Present status. Eur J Surg 2002;168: 260–3.

[12] Chvapil M, Hurych J, Ehrlichova E. The influence of varying oxygen tensions upon proline hydroxylation and the metabolism of collagenous and noncollagenous proteins in skin slices. Hoppe Seylers Z Physiol Chem 1968;349:211–7.

[13] Krueger JK, Rohrich RJ. Clearing the smoke: the scientific rationale for tobacco abstention with plastic surgery. Plast Reconstr Surg 2001;108:1063–73 [discussion: 1074–7].

[14] Goodson III WH, Hunt TK. Wound healing in well-controlled diabetic men. Surg Forum 1984;35:614–6.

[15] Cheung AH, Wong LM. Surgical infections in patients with chronic renal failure. Infect Dis Clin North Am 2001;15:775–96.

[16] Burns J, Pieper B. HIV/AIDS: impact on healing. Ostomy Wound Manage 2000;46:30–40.

[17] Davis PA, Corless DJ, Gazzard BG, et al. Increased risk of wound complications and poor healing following laparotomy in HIV-seropositive and AIDS patients. Dig Surg 1999;16:60–7.

[18] Jeejeebhoy KN. The role of micronutrients in the 1990s. Curr Opin Clin Nutr Metab Care 1998;1:487–9.

[19] Windsor J, Knight G, Hill G. Wound healing response in surgical patients: recent food intake is more important than nutritional status. Br J Surg 1988;75:135–7.

[20] Tibbs MK. Wound healing following radiation therapy: a review. Radiother Oncol 1997;42:99–106.

[21] Grant RA, Cox RW, Kent CM. The effects of gamma irradiation on the structure and reactivity of native and crosslinked collagen fibers. J Anat 1973;115:29–43.

[22] Anstead GM. Steroids, retinoids, and wound healing. Adv Wound Care 1998;11:277–85.

[23] Robson MC, Edstrom LE, Krizek TJ, et al. The efficacy of systemic antibiotics in the treatment of the granulating wound. J Surg Res 1974;16:299–306.

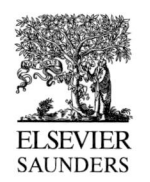

Nutritional Aspects of Care

James C. Fang, DDS, MPH, Desai N. Chirag, DMD, Harry Dym, DDS*

Department of Oral and Maxillofacial Surgery, The Brooklyn Hospital, 121 DeKalb Avenue, Brooklyn, NY 11201, USA

The concept that malnutrition impacts outcomes in surgical patients was shown in 1936; Studley found a 33% mortality rate in patients who experience a postoperative weight loss greater than 20%, compared with 5% for those with a lesser degree of weight loss following gastric resection in patients who develop chronic peptic ulcer disease [1]. Ever since, nutritional support in the surgical and critically ill patient has been recognized as one of the critical components in the perioperative aspect of care. Several recent studies also have delineated the association between degrees of nutritional deficit and poor outcomes in the surgical patient [2–4]. Malnourished surgical patients are associated with an increased risk for morbidity and mortality. Poor nutritional status can compromise the function of many organ systems, including the heart, lungs, kidneys, and gastrointestinal tract (GI) [5]. Immune function and muscle strength also are impaired, leaving these patients more vulnerable to infection and the need for prolonging mechanical ventilation time [6]. Wound healing also is delayed, leading to prolonged surgical recovery [7]. All these factors associated with poor nutrition contribute to a longer hospital stay, higher readmission rates, and markedly increased health care costs [7]. Malnutrition causes the following deleterious consequences:

1) Increased susceptibility to infection
2) Poor wound healing
3) Abnormal nutrient losses through the stool
4) Overgrowth of bacteria in the GI tract
5) Increased frequency of decubitus ulcers

The prevalence of malnutrition among hospitalized patients has been estimated as high as 50% [8]. Approximately 1 in 10 patients experience severe protein-calorie malnutrition [8–10]; therefore, it is the physician's or surgeon's responsibilities to understand the stress response to the injured and critically ill patient and to provide adequate nutritional support. The stress of surgery or trauma increases protein and energy requirements by creating a hypermetabolic, catabolic state. A redistribution of macronutrients (fat, protein, and glycogen) from the labile reserves of adipose tissue and skeletal muscle to more metabolically active tissues, such as liver, bone, and visceral organs, occurs. This response can lead to the onset of protein calorie malnutrition (defined as a negative balance of 100 g of nitrogen and 10,000 kcal within a few days). The rate of development of malnutrition in critically ill patients is a function of preexisting nutritional status and degree of hypermetabolism.

Nutritional assessment in the surgical patient

Nutritional assessment is the evaluation of an individual's nutritional status and nutrient requirements based on the interpretation of clinical information obtained from the patient's medical history, including social history and nutritional history; review of systems; and physical examination, including anthropometric measurements and laboratory data. The goal of a nutritional assessment is to devise an individual unique nutritional plan for each patient. Each critically ill or injured patient has a unique medical history, social history, and nutritional history. An elderly, critically ill, or injured patient also may have comorbid conditions. For example, cancer,

---

* Corresponding author.
E-mail address: hdymdds@yahoo.com (H. Dym).

chronic obstructive pulmonary disease, heart disease, and alcoholism produce additional metabolic challenges and complications. Most times, a young, critically ill, or injured patient may not have these medical conditions previously discussed. Because of the heterogeneity of this patient population, it is difficult to devise nutritional guidelines applicable to all critically ill and injured patients.

History

Before beginning a nutritional assessment, it is necessary to determine which patients require nutritional support. These patients include: those who have had preexisting malnutrition; the healthy, uninjured patient who has been without nutrition for 5 to 7 days; the trauma patient who has an Injury Severity Score greater than 15; a burn patient who has a body surface area burn greater than 20%; and the patient who has severe peritonitis or septicemia [11]. These patients are at risk for malnutrition because of their hypermetabolic state, which is defined as an increase in metabolic rate in excess of the normal metabolic response. This hypermetabolic process leads to a marked increase in energy expenditure and uses protein as an energy source.

A nutritional assessment should begin by an interview with the patient or the patient's family or caregiver who is familiar with the patient's dietary history. A thorough and accurate history of all patients, including medical history, social history, and dietary history is crucial to developing an accurate assessment of the patient's overall status and future needs. The medical history should consist of a review of the patient's past medical history; current medication, including prescription drugs, over-the counter medications, herbal medications, vitamins, minerals and nutritional supplements; and a review of the patient's past surgical history and hospitalizations. The social history includes occupation, sexual history, daily exercise pattern, and marital and family status. In addition, details concerning the duration and frequency of substance use, such as alcohol, tobacco, illegal drugs, and caffeine, are important. The nutrition history should include questions regarding the patient's eating habits, including an approximation of nutrient intake and recent and chronic weight loss [12]. Recent weight loss (5% in the last month or 10% over 6 months) or a current body weight of 80% to 85% (or less) of ideal body weight suggests significant malnutrition [8]. Review of systems should focus on symptoms not diagnoses. One goal of this history is to determine whether any dietary changes have occurred in the patient's life, voluntarily or as a consequence of illness, medication use, or psychologic problems.

Physical examination

The physical examination should be nutritionally oriented and should include selected laboratory tests. The thorough examination should focus on the skin, head, hair, eyes, mouth, nails, abdomen, skeletal muscle, and fat stores. Muscle wasting, especially thenar and temporal muscles, loose or flabby; peripheral edema; hair changes; hepatomegaly; skin rash; glossitis; gingival lesions; pallor; neuropathy; and dementia may indicate malnutrition and nutritional deficiency. Anthropometric measurements, such as midarm muscle circumference, and triceps skinfold measurement, may add information regarding skeletal muscle mass and body-fat stores, respectively. These measures are safe, simple, and inexpensive, but they are not useful in the critically ill patient [13]. The current body weight often is compared with the ideal body weight (IBW) for height to roughly estimate nutritional status. Body mass index (BMI) may also be a useful tool to evaluate nutritional status (Table 1). This index is calculated by weight in kilograms divided by the height in meters squared: BMI = weight (kg)/height (m^2), total lymphocyte count (TLC) = (% lymphocyte × white blood cell [WBC] count)/100.

Biomarkers of nutritional status

Numerous markers exist for testing nutritional status (Table 2); however, no single marker measures nutritional status accurately. Serum albumin levels were studied extensively and found this protein to be an excellent predictor of surgical outcomes when evaluated preoperatively [14–18]. Furthermore, the albumin level was a better predictor of some types of

Table 1
Weight status and classification of nutritional status

Index	Mild	Moderate	Severe	Appropriate w	Overweight	Obese
BMI (kg/m^2)	17–18.5	16–16.9	<16	18.5–24.9	25–29.9	>30

Table 2
Biomarkers to determine level of malnutrition

Index	Mild	Moderate	Severe
Albumin (g/dL)	2.8–3.5	2.1–2.7	<2.1
Transferrin (mg/dL)	151–200	100–150	<100
Prealbumin (mg/dL)	10–15	5–9.9	<5
TLC (per mm^3)	1500–1800	900–1499	<900

morbidity, particular sepsis and major infection in a prospective study by Gibbs and colleagues [16]. The normal range of serum albumin is 3.5 to 5 g/dL. The half-life of albumin is approximately 18 to 21 days and reflects nutritional status over the previous 3 weeks. Albumin is synthesized in and catabolized by the liver. Unfortunately, serum albumin levels decrease with acute stress, overhydration, trauma, surgery, renal loss, hepatic insufficiency, and failure; therefore, in acute setting, albumin is not a reliable nutritional indicator.

Prealbumin, also referred to as transthyretin, is another nutritional status indicator with a half-life of $t^{1/2} = 2$ to 3 days [7], and it is also the least helpful in assessing overall nutritional status because it reflects protein status over past days and weeks. Prealbumin is synthesized by the liver and partly catabolized by the kidneys. Normal serum prealbumin levels range from 16 to 40 mg/dL, but some levels are influenced by many factors, including renal dysfunction, corticosteroid therapy, fluid status, infection, and liver dysfunction.

Transferrin and retinol-binding protein also have been used as markers of nutritional status with half-lives of $t^{1/2} = 8$ to 9 days and $t^{1/2} = 12$ hours, respectively [19]. Serum transferrin levels are influenced by several factors, including liver disease, fluid status, stress, and illness, whereas serum retinol-binding protein levels are affected by vitamin A status. Because transferring also reflects iron status, low transferring should be considered a reliable indication of protein calorie malnutrition only in the setting of normal serum iron.

Measures of immunocompetence

Immune function also can be used to assess nutritional status. Nutritional indices follows:

$$BMI = weight(kg)/height(m^2)$$

$$TLC = (\% \text{ lymphocyte} \times WBC)/100$$

A TLC of less than 3000 mm^3 reflects immunodeficiency [20]. The other is delayed-type hypersensitivity test. In malnutrition, the skin test would be anergic to common skin antigens. Some limitations exist for these two tests, especially for critically ill patients. Sepsis, trauma, and disseminated intravascular coagulopathy also depress immune function.

Caloric and nitrogen balance studies

Several methods to measure calories. One of the most commonly used methods is the Harris-Benedict equation, which can be used to predict basal energy expenditure (BEE), the heat production of basal metabolism in the resting and fasting state:

Man: BEE (Kcal/d) = 66.4 + (13.7 × weight in kg) +(5 × height in cm) − (6.7 × ages in years)

Woman: BEE(Kcal/d) = 655 + (9.6 × weight in kg) +(1.8 × height in cm) − (4.7 × ages in years)

Another simplified predictive equation for calculating BEE is by multiplying weight in kilograms by 24 (kg). Approximation of daily adult basal energy needs (average [AVG] = 1cal/kg/h) can be calculated using the following:

Man: 70 kg AVG, 70 × 24 = 1680

Woman: 58 kg AVG, 58 × 24 = 1390

These equations provide a reliable estimate of the energy requirement in approximately 80% of hospitalized patients [8]; however, the actual caloric needs in the hypermetabolic or stress patient may be underestimated. Adjustments, therefore, in the BEE have been proposed (Table 3) [21]. For example, correction factors for the skeletal trauma and soft tissue trauma are 1.2 and 1.14, respectively [20]. The adjusted BEE may overestimate the daily energy requirement of the stress patient by 20% to 60% [21]. For this reason, the more accurate method to measure energy requirement is indirect calorimetry, a tech-

Table 3
Correction factor used in calculation of BEE

Patient condition	Correction factor
Fever (for each °C above the normal body temperature)	1.1
Mild stress	1.2
Moderate stress	1.4
Severe stress	1.6

nique that measures the whole body oxygen consumption (VO$_2$) and carbon dioxide production (VCO$_2$) by using a specialize instrument called a metabolic cart to calculate resting energy expenditure. Several limitations of indirect calorimetry exist. First, the equipment is expensive and requires specialized trained personnel to operate. In addition, the oxygen sensor in most metabolic carts is not reliable at FiO$_2$ or greater than 50%. As a result, indirect calorimetry is reserved only for patients who fail to respond adequately to the estimated nutritional needs; patients who have single- or multiple-organ dysfunction and are in need of prolonged intensive care unit care and artificial nutritional support; mechanically ventilated patients who have acute respiratory failure induced by artificial nutrition on the cardiocirculatory and respiratory systems; and patients who need monitoring of VO$_2$ during weaning from mechanical ventilation [21,22].

Nitrogen balance study provides an inexpensive, effective way to assess protein requirements, calculated by subtracting the total excreted nitrogen from the total dietary nitrogen intake over a 24-hour period. A positive nitrogen balance, typically in the range of 2 to 4 g of nitrogen per day is desired but is difficult to achieve in the critically ill patient.

Caloric and energy requirement

The goal of nutritional support in the critically ill and injured patient is maintenance not repletion. Energy requirements should be obtained from carbohydrates and lipids. Carbohydrates are stored as a glycogen in the human body, approximately, 100 g of glycogen is stored in the liver and 200 to 250 g of glycogen is stored in the heart and muscle tissue. Glycogen in the liver is available to maintain to the glucose level of the blood, whereas glycogen in the heart and muscle is available only for muscle energy. Glucose is a principal energy source in carbohydrates of the human body. The energy content of glucose is 3.7 kcal/g. Daily intake of carbohydrates is necessary to ensure the proper functioning of the central nervous system and erythrocytes, which are dependent on glucose as their principal fuel source. Excess intake of carbohydrates, however, can produce adverse effects, such as lipogenesis and excess production of carbon dioxide.

Lipids are the most concentrated source of heat and energy and they are stored as triglycerides in adipose tissues and represent the major endogenous energy source. The energy content of the lipid is about 9 kcal/g and the triglycerides are composed of a

Table 4
Recommended daily protein intake

Clinical condition	Protein requirements (g/kg IBW/d)
Normal	0.8
Metabolic "stress" (illness/injury)	1.0–1.5
Acute renal failure (undialyzed)	0.8–1.0
Hemodialysis	1.2–1.4
Peritoneal dialysis	1.3–1.5

glycerol molecule linked to three fatty acids. The only essential fatty acid is linoleic acid and providing 0.5% of the dietary fatty acids as linoleic acid can prevent an essential fatty acid disorder [21]. The minimum calorie requirement that should be delivered as linoleic acid to prevent essential fatty acid deficiency is 1% to 2% when total parenteral nutrition (TPN) is used [23].

Protein requirements

Protein serves an important role in building new body tissues, maintaining body structure, producing essential compounds, such as enzymes and hormones, regulating water balance, maintaining blood neutrality, and providing energy. Amino acids are the building structure for proteins and are composed of 10 essential amino acids and 10 nonessential acids. Liver is the primary site to regulate plasma amino acid. The total body protein is present mostly in skeletal muscle. Daily protein turnover is approximately 3% of total body protein. The primary site of turnover is in the GI tract where shed enterocytes and secreted digestive enzymes are lost regularly. The normal protein intake requirement is 0.8 to 1.0 g/kg/d, whereas the hypermetabolic protein intake requirement is 1.2 g to 2.0 g/kg/d. In trauma patients, no published studies have demonstrated any benefits of providing more than 1.5 g/kg of protein (Table 4) [20]. The purpose of providing protein nutritional support is not to provide energy but to provide protein to be used for protein synthesis.

Micronutrients

Micronutrients consist of vitamins and minerals. Vitamins are divided further into water-soluble and fat-soluble vitamins. The water-soluble vitamins include vitamin C, the vitamin B complex, and biotin. Vitamins A, D, E, and K constitute the fat-soluble vitamins. The water-soluble vitamins generally serve as coenzymes in energy and protein metabolism. On the other hand, the fat-soluble vitamins play an important role in various cellular functions, including cellular differentiation and proliferation, skeletal formation, immune function, antioxidant activity, and blood coagulation. Minerals are categorized further as macrominerals and microminerals, also called traced minerals. Major minerals consist of major electrolytes, calcium, sodium, potassium, magnesium, phosphorus, and sulfur. They constitute approximately 0.01% of total body weight [24]. Microminerals include iron, zinc, copper, selenium, iodine, manganese, molybdenum, fluoride, and chromium. These trace elements exist in less than one part per million of body weight [24].

Soluble vitamins

Vitamin C (ascorbic acid) is an important antioxidant vitamin. Not only does it play an important role in collagen formation as a cofactor in the hydroxylation of praline and lysine residues, it also participates in other enzyme functions, such as in biosynthesis of bile acids, carnitine, and catecholamines. Its effects, moreover, on immune function include improved polymorphonuclear cell adherence, delivery and motility, increased antibody production, and enhanced lymphoproliferative response [25]. Furthermore, it regenerates other antioxidants, such as vitamin E, flavonoids, and glutathione [21]. The normal serum vitamin C level is between 0.6 and 2 mg/dL [21] and WBC ascorbic acid concentration is a more accurate measure of a vitamin C nutritional state [26]. Serum vitamin C levels less than 0.1 mg/dL reflect a state of nutritional adequacy. The recommend daily allowances (RDA) for vitamin C is 75 mg/d and 90 mg/d for women and men, respectively. Deficiency of vitamin C leads to impaired wound healing, weakness, scurvy, and decreased resistance to infection [24,27]. In one study, it was found that plasma vitamin C levels are depressed in critically patients in relation to severity of illness [28]. The recommended daily requirements of vitamin C in enteral and parenteral nutritional support are 60 and 100 mg, respectively [21]. Optimal supplementation should not exceed 200 mg/d [24].

Vitamin B complexes include thiamin (B_1), riboflavin (B_2), niacin (B_3), pantothenic acid (B_5), pyridoxine (B_6), folic acid (B_9) and cobalamin (B_{12}).

Each vitamin B has its own unique role in metabolism. They are all essential cofactors in many metabolic pathways. Increased energy and protein metabolism during the stress response results in an increased need for B complex vitamins [24]. Thiamine plays important roles not only in carbohydrate metabolism but also in nerve transmission. Deficiency of thiamine leads to beriberi, neuropathy, and cardiac dysfunction [27,29]. In alcoholic patients, the deficiency may have central nervous manifestations known as Wernicke's encephalopathy, consisting of horizontal nystagmus, ophthalmoplegia, cerebella ataxia, and mental impairment [29]. When an additional loss of memory and a confabulatory psychosis occurs, the syndrome is known as Wernicke-Korsakoff syndrome [29]. The total body store of thiamine, mainly in the form of thiamine pyrophosphate, is approximately 30 mg [29]. In ICU patients, if thiamine is not supplemented for 10 days, the endogenous thiamine store is depleted [21]. The RDA for vitamin B_1 is 1.2 mg/d for men and 1.1 mg/d for women [28]. One of the most reliable laboratory tests is the measurement of whole blood or erythrocyte transketolase activity before and after the addition of thiamine pyrophosphate (TPP) [21]. An increase in enzyme activity greater than 25% after the addition of TPP reflects thiamine deficiency [21]. B_1 can also be measured in the serum and urine to detect the deficiency [29]. The recommended daily requirements for vitamin B_1 in enteral and parenteral nutritional support are 1.4 mg and 3 mg, respectively [21,30].

Riboflavin (B_2) plays an important role for the metabolism of fat, carbohydrate, and protein. In addition, it is a component of oxidation-reduction processes. Deficiency of riboflavin primarily manifests as mucocutaneous lesions of the mouth, including angular stomatitis, cheilosis, atrophic glossitis, and pharyngitis, and in the skin as seborrhea and genital dermatitis [27,29]. The RDA for riboflavin is 1.1 to 1.3 mg. The recommended daily requirements for vitamin B_2 in enteral and parenteral nutritional support is 1.6 mg and 3.6 mg, respectively [21,30].

Niacin (B_3) is a collective term and refers to nicotinic acid and nicotinamide and their biologically active derivatives. Niacin serves crucial roles in pentose, steroid, and fatty acid biosynthesis. Moreover, niacin acts a coenzyme in glycolysis, protein metabolism, and the Krebs cycle. Furthermore, niacin is involved in DNA repair and calcium mobilization. The RDA for niacin is 16 niacin equivalents per day for men and 14 niacin equivalents per day for women [29]. One niacin is equivalent to 60 mg tryptophan because the amino acid tryptophan can be converted to niacin with an efficiency of 60:1 by weight [29]. Deficiency of niacin causes pellagra, which is found primarily in alcoholics in the United States [27,29]. The diagnosis of niacin deficiency is based on low levels of urinary metabolites 2-methyl nicotinamide and 2-pyridone [29]. The recommended daily requirements for vitamin B_3 in enteral and parenteral nutritional support are 18 mg and 40 mg, respectively [30].

Pyridoxine (B_6) refers to a family of compounds, including pyridoxine, pyridoxal, pyridoxamine, and their 5′-phosphate derivatives. Vitamin B_6 is required for amino acid metabolism and protein synthesis [24] and also is involved in heme and neurotransmitter synthesis and in the metabolism of glycogen, lipids, steroids, and sphingoid bases and several vitamins, including the conversion of tryptophan to niacin [29]. The biologic half-life of vitamin B_6 is 25 days and the RDA for vitamin B_6 is from 1.3 to 1.7 mg/d [29]. Deficiency of vitamin B_6 leads to symptoms similar to deficiency of B_2. The severe form of vitamin B_6 deficiency manifests as generalized weakness, irritability, peripheral neuropathy, and convulsion [27,29]. The diagnosis of vitamin B_6 is based on low plasma 5′-pyridoxal phosphate values (<20 nmol/L) [29]. Other laboratory tests, including erythrocyte levels of 5′-pyridoxal phosphate, plasma levels of pyridoxal, and urinary levels of 4-pyridoxix acid can be used to detect the deficiency of vitamin B_6 [29]. The recommended daily requirements for vitamin B_6 in enteral and parenteral nutritional support are 2 mg and 4 mg, respectively [21,31].

Pantothenic acid (B_5) is a component of coenzyme A and phosphopantetheine. Pantothenic acid functions in the oxidation of fatty acids and carbohydrates for energy production and the synthesis of fatty acids, ketones, cholesterol, phospholipids, steroid hormones, and amino acids. The RDA for vitamin B_5 is not established; however, the adequate intake (AI) is set at 5 mg/d for adult men and women [31]. Deficiency of B_5 occurs rarely but leads to nonspecific symptoms, including GI disturbance, depression, muscle cramps, parethesia, ataxia, and hypoglycemia [27,29]. Urinary levels of pantothenic acid can be used to detect deficiency [32,33]. The recommended daily requirements for vitamin B_5 in enteral and parenteral nutritional support are 5 mg and 15 mg, respectively [21,30].

Cobalamin (B_{12}) is a complex organometallic compound and it plays vital roles in formation of mature erythrocyte and folate metabolism [34]. Cobalamin is an essential cofactor for two enzymes in human cells: methionine synthase, which catalyzes the conversion of homocysteine to methionine, and methylmalonyl-CoA synthase, which catalyzed the conversion of methylmalonyl CoA to succinyl CoA. Deficiency of cobalamin leads to pernicious anemia, neurologic abnormalities, including peripheral neuropathies, gait disturbance, memory loss, and psychiatric symptoms [27,34]. Certain medications also can cause deficiency in addition to malabsorption in those who are vegetarians and lack a complete diet [31]. About 2 mg cobalamin is stored in the liver, and another 2 mg is stored elsewhere in the body [34]. The RDA for cobalamin is 2.4 ug/d for men and women [31]. Cobalamin deficiency can be detected by serum cobalamin levels. If levels are less than 100 pg/mL, it is a clinically significant deficiency. The recommended daily requirements for vitamin B_{12} in enteral and parenteral nutritional support are 3 ug and 5 ug, respectively [21,30].

Folic acid (B_9) is the common name for pterylmonglutamic acid and is responsible for numerous pathways, especially those of amino acid and nucleotide metabolism, and DNA synthesis. In normal individuals, the total body has about 5 to 20 mg of folic acid in various body stores, half in the liver [34]. The RDA for folic acid is 200 mg for men and women [31]. Deficiency of folic acid manifests megalobalstic anemia [27]. Diarrhea, cheilosis, and glossitis also are seen [34]. Several studies have shown that the requirement for folic acid during critical illness is increased [35,36]. Serum levels of folic acid can detect folic acid deficiency. Values less than and equal to 4 ng/mL are considered to be diagnostic of folate deficiency [34]. Measurement of red blood cell (RBC) folate levels provides a better index of folate store than serum folate because it is not subject to short-term fluctuations in folate intake [34]. Medications, such as inhibitors of dihydrofolate reductase, are one of the common causes for folate deficiency. For example, methotrexate can impair DNA metabolism and produce folate deficiency [34]. Chronic alcoholics also may have folic acid deficiency. The recommended daily requirement for vitamin B_9 in enteral and parenteral nutritional support is 400 ug [21,30].

Biotin plays an important role in gluconeogenesis and fatty acid synthesis. The vitamin biotin also functions in the metabolism of specific amino acid (eg, leucine) and serves as a CO_2 carrier on the surface of cytosolic and mitochondrial carboxylase enzymes. The RDA for vitamin biotin is not established; however, the AI is set at 30 ug/d for adult men and women [31,37]. Deficiency of biotin is rare and has been demonstrated with prolong parenteral nutrition with biotin supplment and results in mental changes, parethesia, anorexia, nausea, hair loss, and dermatitis [27,31]. Urinary levels of biotin and its metabolite especially 3-hydroyxisovaleric acid can be used to detect and monitor the status of biotin [38]. The recommended daily requirement for vitamin biotin in enteral and parenteral nutritional support is 60 ug [21,30].

Fat-soluble vitamins

Besides playing a well-known role in vision, vitamin A is important for cellular differentiation, for the functioning of the immune systems, and for the iron use [24,39,40]. Vitamin A also helps form and maintain healthy teeth, skeletal and soft tissue, mucous membranes, and skin [40]. Low circulating vitamin levels are associated with adaptive immunity and with diminishing function of neutrophils, macrophages, and natural killer cells [39]. Consequently, vitamin A plays a role in preventing and treating infection [24]. Liver is the major storage site for vitamin A and the RDA for vitamin A is 800 ug retinol equivalents (RE) for women and 1000 ug RE for men [31]. One RE is defined as 1 ug of retinol. Deficiency of vitamin A leads to symptoms, such as hyperkeratotic skin lesions, night blindness, dryness of the eyes, xerosis, and Bitôt spots, which are white patches of keratinized epithelium appearing on the sclera [27,29]. Measurement of serum retinol can be used to detect deficiency. Other tests, including tests of dark adapatation, impression cytology of the conjuctiva, or measurement of body storage pools, may also be used [29]. The recommended daily requirement for vitamin A in enteral and parenteral nutritional support is 1000 ug [21,30].

Vitamin D exists in several forms and each with a different level of activity. Calciferol is the most active form of vitamin D. Vitamin D plays a crucial role in maintenance of calcium homeostasis and does not require dietary supplementation as long as adequate exposure to sunlight exists. Once vitamin D_3 is produced in the skin or consumed in food, it requires chemical conversion in the liver and kidney to form 1,25 dihydroxy vitamin D, the physiologically active form of vitamin D [41,42]. The RDA for vitamin D is not established; however, the AI is from 5 ug/d to 15 ug/d for adult men and women depending on age [31]. Deficiency of vitamin D leads to rickets and ostomalacia. Measurement of serum vitamin D can be used to monitor and detect the deficiency. The recommended daily requirement for vitamin D in enteral and parenteral nutritional supports is 10 ug [21,30].

Vitamin E is a mixtures of tocopherols and tocotrinols. Alpha-tocopherol (α-tocopherol) is one of the most active forms of vitamin E in humans. Besides its well-known role in antioxidant activity, vitamin E also has been shown to play a role in immune function and in DNA repair and cell-regulating effects by maintenance of protein thiol [24,29]. The RDA for vitamin E is 10 mg α-tocoherol equivalents (TE) per day [31]. Deficiency of vitamin E is rare and may lead to neuropathy and hemolysis [27]. Several studies have shown that vitamin E levels are low during critically ill periods [42,43]. The laboratory diagnosis of vitamin E deficiency is made by low blood levels of α-tocopherol [24,29]. Values less than 5 ug/ml or α-tocopherol per gram of total lipids ratio less than 0.8 mg indicate deficiency [24,29]. The recommended daily requirement for vitamin D in enteral and parenteral nutritional support is 10 mg [21,30].

Vitamin K exists in two natural forms: phylloquinone, which is obtained from vegetable and animal sources, and menaquinone, which is synthesized by bacterial flora and found in hepatic tissue [29]. Vitamin K has an important role in the coagulation pathway especially for Factors II (prothrombin), VII, IX, and X. It may also have roles in bone mineralization and cell growth [44,45]. The RDA for vitamin K is 70 ug/d for adults [31]. Deficiency of vitamin K leads to hemorrhage. Medications, such as broad-spectrum antibiotics, may precipitate the deficiency of vitamin K by reducing gut bacteria and by inhibiting the metabolism of vitamin K. The prothrombin time and International Normalized Ratio can be used to detect and monitor the vitamin K deficiency. Reduced levels of clotting factors can be used to make diagnosis of vitamin K deficiency. In addition, under-carboxylated prothrombin and low gla levels in urine indicate vitamin K deficiency [29]. The recommended daily requirements for vitamin K in enteral and parenteral nutritional support are 100 ug and 200 ug, respectively [21,30].

Macrominerals

Macrominerals not only consist of major electrolytes (potassium and sodium), but also include calcium, magnesium, phosphorous, and sulfur. The goal of macromineral supplementation is to maintain adequate circulating plasma levels; therefore, judicious monitoring of major electrolytes, calcium, magnesium, phosphorous is necessary. The physiology and biologic processes that require macrominerals include neuromuscular excitation, enzymatic activation, blood coagulation, and membrane permeability.

For example, calcium participates in blood coagulation, neuromuscular transmission, smooth muscle contraction, and maintaining the structure integrity of the bony skeleton. Deficiency of macrominerals is present frequently in the critically ill. Medication nutrient interactions are predominant reasons, but other reasons, such as large GI losses, acid base imbalances, malnutrition, fever, and increased metabolism, also may contribute to the macromineral deficiency. In the critically ill patients, proper management of macrominerals is important because it impacts on nutritional adequacy, hospital costs, and patient outcome.

Microminerals

Zinc plays a fundamental role in cellular growth and replication, protein synthesis, immune function, wound healing, and metabolism of carbohydrates [24,29,46]. The body contains approximately 2 g of zinc, which is stored in liver, prostate, pancreas, bone, and brain [29]. The RDA for zinc is 15 mg for men and 12 mg for women [31]. A deficiency in zinc may lead to impaired immune function, night blindness, and decreased taste sensation [24,29,47]. The diagnosis of zinc deficiency usually is made by a serum zinc level of less than 12 $u$mol/L. The recommended daily requirements for zinc in enteral and parenteral nutritional support are 15 mg and 4 mg, respectively [21,30]. Additional supplementation of zinc is controversial for pharmacologic effect on wound healing and immunity because of limited supportive evidence of benefits [24].

Copper is required in the formation of hemoglobin, RBCs, and bones [29], and plays an important role in wound healing, melanin synthesis, central nervous system function, and the scavenging of superoxide radicals [29]. The body contains 50 to 120 mg of copper stored in the liver [29]. The RDA for copper is 1.5 to 3 mg [29]. Deficiency of copper is rare and is attributed to disturbances in the metabolism of its carrier protein ceruloplasmin. The diagnosis of copper deficiency usually is made by low serum levels of copper (<65 ug/dL) and low ceruloplasmin levels (<18 mg/dL) [24,29]. The recommended daily requirements for copper in enteral and parenteral nutritional support are 3mg and 0.5 mg, respectively [21,30]. Little evidence supports additional supplementation of copper for critically ill patients [24].

Iron plays a central role in carrying oxygen as a component of the heme molecule, and is a vital element in the function of all cells and in iron-containing enzymes. Iron in the human body is bound primarily to the proteins: hemoglobin, ferritin, and transferrin [48]. Little iron is found circulating in plasma as free and unbound [21,48]. Excessive amounts of unbound iron produce systemic toxicity in which it participates in chemical reactions that generate free radicals [21,48]. Anemia occurring in those patients who are critically ill is a common result of derangement of iron metabolism [49]. Other factors, such as increased destruction or impaired production of erythrocytes and blood loss because of frequent diagnostic testing may contribute to patients developing anemia [24]. The recommended daily requirements for iron in enteral and parenteral nutritional support are 10 mg and 1 mg, respectively [21,30]. However, a reduced serum iron level in a critically ill patient should not prompt iron replacement therapy unless evidence of total-body iron deficiency exists [21,24,47]. Deficiency of total-iron can be detected with serum iron, total-iron binding capacity, serum ferritin, and percent saturation. Values of ferritin less than 15 ug/L indicate iron deficiency [48].

Selenium is a component of enzyme glutathione peroxidase, which is one of the important endogenous antioxidant enzymes. Glutathione peroxidase serves a role in protecting proteins, cell membranes, lipids, and nucleic acid from oxidant molecules. The RDA for selenium is 55 ug and 70 ug for women and men, respectively [29]. Selenium during critically ill periods may be deficient because of an increase in use, insufficient intake, and an increased cutaneous loss [21,24,50]. A small pilot study in Germany has shown selenium supplementation may be beneficial for critically ill [51] patients. Selenium deficiency can be detected by measuring serum selenium level [21,24]. The recommended daily requirements for iron in enteral and parenteral nutritional support are 200 ug and 75 ug, respectively [21,30].

Immunonutrition

Immnunutrion is one of the most prominent areas of controversy when discussing nutritional support in recent years. Various compounds are believed to be immune-enhancing formulas or immune-modulating formulas, including arginine, glutamine, nucleic acid, and omega-3 fatty acids [7,20]. The concepts behind these formulas is to protect and stimulate the immune system with the goal of reducing infectious complications, decreasing multiorgan failure, decreasing time on mechanical ventilation, and decreasing length of hospital or intensive-care stay [7,20]. A review article by Heyland has concluded that immunonutrition may decrease infectious complications rates in elective surgical patients [52]. However, in critically ill patients, immunonutrition is not associated with any apparent clinical benefits and may be harmful. Other studies also suggest that immunonutrition may decrease infectious complication in GI surgical and trauma patients [53–55]. Consensus guidelines that have been developed by numerous clinical investigators and published in 2001 suggest that immunonutrition is beneficial for moderate to severely malnourished patients undergoing elective GI surgery, patients who exhibit an injury severity score of 18 or greater, and trauma patients who exhibit an abdominal trauma index of 20 or more [56]. Despite many randomized human studies, clinical studies of immunonutrition have yet to identify their optimal effect and role in therapy. More clinical research is needed before more precise guidelines can be recommended.

Timing

Established consensus guidelines do not exist as to when to begin nutritional support. The goal for nutritional support is not to prevent morbidity or mortality only, but it also attenuates the hypermetabolic response to injury, reduces the rate of infectious complications, and maintains the integrity of the intestinal mucosa [57]. For the most part, nutritional support for a well-nourished perioperative patient or the less severely injured patient is not routinely indicated. The body can compensate for inadequate nutrient intake by breakdown of glycogen stores, gluconeogenesis, peripheral lipolysis, and amino acid oxidation from muscle stores. For well-nourished adults, inadequate oral intake of 7 to 14 days is a widely accepted cut-off prompting nutritional intervention. Infants and children have proportionately lower reserves of body protein, carbohydrate, and fat than adults and also have increased metabolic needs. As a result, insufficient oral intake for 3 to 7 days is a more suitable trigger for intervention in children. Any variation, such as advanced age, major injury, or the presence of comorbidities can deplete the patient's nutritional reserve more drastically and quickly. Although this type of patient needs adequate nutritional support, the optimal timing has not been elucidated. Indications for nutritional support are patients who cannot maintain an oral diet for a prolonged period or someone who has preexisting malnutrition. Patients who are not hemodynamically stable should not receive nutritional support. One study has shown that early feeding during the shock state can contribute to mesenteric ischemia, infarction, and perforation [58]. The benefits of early feeding in hypermetabolic patients have not been well studied. The heterogeneity of these conditions and the individual patient's varied metabolic response make the study designs problematic and flawed. Moore and colleagues were the first to demonstrate that early enteral feeding reduced the septic complication as compared with a control group who received total parenteral nutrition (TPN) [59]. In addition, Lewis and colleagues did a meta-analysis to demonstrate that early enteral feeding reduced infectious complication as compared with nothing by mouth after abdominal surgery [60]. Furthermore, TPN was found to decrease complications in severely malnourished populations only [61]. Although the early initiation of nutritional support has some benefits, it remains unclear when to initiate nutritional support. Most clinicians agree that early feeding in the severely injured patient is favorable and justified.

Enteral nutrition

The term enteral refers to feeding by way of the gut and hence includes normal eating, but in the present context implies the infusion of formula by way of a tube into the upper GI tract. Indications for enteral nutritional support are inability to ingest food normally, obstruction of GI tract if access can be placed below obstruction, impairment of digestion or absorption, physiologic deterrents to food intake, protein-energy malnutrition, and psychiatric illness [62]. Potential contraindications for enteral nutritional support include complete gastric or intestinal obstruction if access cannot be placed distal to obstruction, ileus, high-output enteric fistula (>500 mL/d), moderate to severe acute pancreatitis, severe diarrhea or vomiting, and refusal of nutrition support by the patient or the patient's legal guardian [53,62,63].

Moore and colleagues have demonstrated that enteral feeding has decreased septic complications when compared with TPN in trauma patients [59]. These results have been supported by another study that Kudsk and colleagues published in 1992, which randomized 98 patients who exhibited an abdominal trauma index of at least 15 to receive enteral or parenteral feeding within 24 hours of injury [64]. Furthermore, Braunschweig and colleagues performed a meta-analysis on 27 studies involving 1828 patients [65]. These aggregate studies confirmed a significantly lower risk for infection with enteral nutrition than with TPN. These studies clearly demonstrated that enteral nutrition is the preferred route where feasible because the digestive, absorptive, and immunologic barrier functions of the GI tract have been preserved [66,67]. In addition, cost of enteral nutrition, which is about one tenth of the cost of parenteral nutrition [67], offers additional benefit.

Numerous routes exist to administer enteral nutrition and each has its own benefits and risks. Complications of nasogastric tube feeding include (1) erosive tissue damage—nasopharyngeal, erosions, pharyngitis, sinsitis, and gastrointestinal (GI) tract perforation ; (2) hyperglycemia; (3) pulmonary aspiration; and (4) GI complications—nausea, vomiting, and diarrhea. Nasogastric tubes are chosen when the stomach is intact and empties normally in a short-term (weeks) clinical situation [30]; in addition, the patient must have a normal gag reflex accompanied by good mental status [62]. The nasogastric tube extends from the nose and empties into stomach. The position of the nasogastric tube is confirmed by injecting air and auscultating, aspirating gastric acid, or by chest radiograph. Advantages include bolus or intermittent feeding with the ability to accept high osmotic loads and prevent infection [62]. The potential complications are aspiration and ulceration of nasal and esophageal tissues [30].

The nasojejunal tube also may be used and it extends from the nose and then by way of the pylorus into the duodenum with or without the aids of fluoroscopy or endoscopic loop [30], with its position verified by abdominal radiograph. Indications for its use are patients who are at risk for aspiration or who have poor gag reflexes and those patients who have gastroparesis or delayed gastric emptying [62]. The nasojejunal tube is also used in short-term feeding but requires a continuous drip with a pump, and its most common complication is diarrhea [30].

If enteral feeding is required for more than 3 to 4 weeks, other modes of enteral feeding tubes should be considered. Surgically placed gastrostomy tubes or nonsurgically placed by way of percutaneous endoscopic gastrostomy (PEG) tubes may be indicated for patients who have swallowing disorders or patients who have impaired small-bowel absorption requiring continuous drip [62]. Potential complications include aspiration, irritation around tube exit site, peritoneal leak, and balloon migration and obstruction of pylorus [62]. When patients have impaired gastric emptying, and require long-term feedings, a surgically placed jujunostomy tube or nonsurgically by way of percutaneous endoscopic jejunstomy tube may be indicated [30,62].

Enteral feeding products

Current enteral feeding products are divided into four categories: blenderized formulas, nutritionally complete commercial formulas, chemically defined formulas, and modular formulas [8]. Blenderized and nutritionally complete commercial formulas are a component of polymeric formulas. These polymeric formulas contain intact proteins, carbohydrates, variable fat contents, trace elements, and macronutrients. In addition, they require an intact, normal GI function [8,63]. Caloric distribution of blenderized formulas should parallel that of a normal diet [8]. Nutritionally complete commercial formulas, known as standard enteral diets are convenient, sterile, and low in cost. Several formulas, such as Ensure, Jevity, and Glucerna, are available for and suitable for lactose-deficiency patients and are recommended for patients experiencing minimal metabolic stress [63].

Chemically defined formulas, known as elemental diets, are defined as nutrients that are provided in predigested and readily absorbed form [8,63]. They are useful in malabsorption or maldigestion patients, pancreatic insufficiency patients, or massive bowel resection patients [62]. In addition, they are more expensive than nutritionally complete commercial formulas and are also hyperosmolar, which may cause cramping and diarrhea [63]. Modular formulas, such as ProMod and Microlipid, are designed to provide nutritional support in specific clinical situations; for example, patients who are in renal failure may need ProMod for additional protein nutritional support.

Selecting the appropriate enteral formula is important. Osmolality affects the patient's ability to tolerate the formula [62]. High osmolality (> 1000 mOsm/kg) means a hypertonic formula which should be infused into the stomach to take advantage of the dilutional effects of the gastric secretion to prevent diarrhea [68]. Most enteral formulas are well-tolerated with osmolality ranging from 300 to 700 mOsm/kg. The osmolality of the enteral formulas is determined by the most abundant nutrient, which usually is a carbohydrate [68]. Carbohydrates are also a determinant in caloric density; therefore, osmolality is related directly to caloric density. Most enteral feeding formulas contain 1 kcal/mL, which is also low osmolality. Although some enteral feeding formulas have 2 kcal/mL and are appropriate for patients who experience increased caloric needs or patients who develop fluid restriction. The renal solute load also should be considered and if enteral feeding formulas contain high renal solute loads, hydration status should be monitored carefully. The protein density of enteral feeding formulas is another useful criterion in selecting enteral formulas depending on the patient's nutritional status and disease state.

Enteral feeding protocol

Current recommendations for enteral feeding protocol are that feedings should be started with full-strength formula, begun at a slow rate, and steadily increased to reduce the risk for microbial contamination and to achieve full nutrient intake earlier [8,68,69]. Conservative initiation and advancement rates are reserved for patients who are critically ill, those who have not been fed for some time, and those who are receiving high-osmolality or calorie-dense formula [8]. Two types of enteral feeding protocols have been categorized: bolus feeding and continuous infusion. Bolus feedings are used primarily in patients who have nasogastric or gastrostomy feeding tubes. The feeding rate usually starts at 50 mL every 4 hours and increases in 50-mL increments until the intake goal is reached. The residual gastric volume should be measured every 4 hours before the next feeding bolus is administered and if the residual volume is greater than 50% of the previous bolus, the next feeding should be withheld. Approximately 30 mL of water should be used to flush the feeding tube to prevent the tube occlusion. Tracheobronchial aspiration can be prevented by elevation of the patient's head to between 30° and 45° during feeding and from 1 to 2 hours after each feeding. The diagnosis of tracheal aspiration can be tested by using a glucose oxidase reagent strip [68]. If a glucose concentration is greater than 20 mg/dL, aspiration is indicated. Methylene blue (1 mg/L) added to the feeding formulas also can be used to detect aspiration [68]. Continuous infusion is indicated when the patient has nasojejunal, gastorjejunal, or jujunal feeding tubes. Feedings are initiated at 20 mL/h and increased in 20-ml/h increments every 4 hours until the desire goal is reached; again, 30 mL of water should be used to flush the feeding tube every 4 hours.

Complications of enteral feeding include tube occlusion, aspiration, and diarrhea. Tube occlusion can be avoided by flushing with 30 mL of water every 4 hours. If partial obstruction occurs, warm water can be injected into the tube, resolving the obstruction in 30% of cases [68]. If the obstruction still does not resolve, pancreatic enzyme with sodium bicarbonate can be applied to relieve the obstruction in 70% of cases [70,71]. If the above-stated two methods do not relieve the obstruction, then the tube should be replaced. Aspiration may be reduced by elevating the head of bed to 45° [72]. Glucose test strips and methylene blue added to the enteral feeding can be used to detect aspiration. Aspiration rates between postpyloric and gastric routes are the same [73–75]. Diarrhea, occurring commonly in enteral feeding, is caused by many factors, such as medications that contain sorbitol, hyperosmolar formulas, a diet that is high in fat content, or the presence of components not tolerated by the patient [8]. If diarrhea is determined to be caused by the high feeding rates or strength of enteral feedings, the rate or strength should be reduced. If no improvement occurs, a different formula should be used.

Parenteral nutrition

Parenteral nutrition is administered intravenously. Partial parenteral nutrition supplies only part of the patient's daily nutritional requirements, supplementing oral intake. Many hospitalized patients receive dextrose or amino acid solutions by this method as part of their routine care. TPN supplies all of the patient's daily nutritional requirements. Hypertonic parenteral nutrition solutions should be infused into a large central vein to reduce the risk for intimal damage from the catheter and infusate. The catheter tip must be in a blood vessel with high blood flow that causes rapid dilution thereby reducing the risk for thrombophlebitis. A peripheral vein may be used for short periods, but longer periods of use with concentrated solutions can lead readily to thrombosis; therefore, central venous access is usually required. TPN is used not only in the hospital for long-term administration but also at home (home TPN), enabling many persons who have lost small-bowel function to lead useful lives. Some indications for peripheral TPN are as follows:

Nutritional status not severely compromised
Patient able to tolerate some nutrition orally or internally
Recovery time predicted to be short
Good venous access

Some indications for central TPN are as follows:

Poor nutritional status
Patient unable to tolerate any nutrition internally
Expected prolonged need of nutritional support
Poor peripheral venous access

Total intravenous nutrition necessitates considerable clinical and pharmaceutical expertise and laboratory support to minimize biochemical, bacteriologic, and surgical complications. Infusates must be prepared aseptically. Experienced nursing care must be available to resolve problems related to the catheter, and the patient must be monitored closely.

Intravenous nutrient solutions

TPN requires water (30–40 mL/kg/d) and energy (30–60 kcal/kg/d), depending on energy expenditure, and amino acids (1–3 g/kg/d), depending on the degree of catabolism. These requirements and those for vitamins and minerals in adult patients are summarized in Table 5.

Dextrose solutions

The standard nutritional support regimen uses carbohydrates to supply approximately 70% of the daily nonprotein caloric requirements. These caloric requirements are provided by dextrose solutions which are available in 5%, 10%, 20%, 50%, and 70% strengths yielding between 170 and 2380 kcal/L of energy. Glucose is the sole monosaccharide used for intravenous nutrition. A solution with a glucose concentration of more than 12.5% is too hyperosmolar for peripheral use, whereas a concentration of up to 40% can be administered by way of a central line. The recommended amount of glucose to be infused is from 10 to 20 g/kg/d. Urine must be closely monitored for glucose spillage. Patients, who experience glucosuria, such as those who are infected or stressed, may benefit from the addition of insulin to the intravenous mixture (one unit of regular insulin per 10 g of glucose).

Amino acid solutions

Amino acid solutions are mixed together with the dextrose solutions to provide the daily protein requirements. The range in adults is from 0.5 to 3.5 g/kg/d. Blood urea, nitrogen, and albumin should be monitored. To obtain information on recent protein synthesis, a serum prealbumin, fibronectin, or retinol-binding protein can be measured.

L-amino acids are preferred to D-amino acids because they are more effective in maintaining nitrogen balance and protein synthesis. Nitrogen balance studies allow the clinician to ensure that the protein intake is at a safe level. The balance is the difference between nitrogen intake and nitrogen losses in the urine (as urinary urea), stools, and sweat. Losses also can occur through the skin in burn patients. Starvation and infections result in a state of negative balance and rapid growth a positive balance.

Lipid emulsions

Parenteral lipids provide high energy in a small volume with a low osmolar load and also are a source of the essential fatty acids, linoleic and linolenic acids. Fat emulsion solutions are available as 10% or 20% preparations, with osmolalities of 280 mosmol/kg and 330 mosmol/kg, respectively. They are derived from soybean, safflower, or cottonseed oil, with the fat mainly present as triglyceride. The 20% emulsion provides approximately 2 kcal/mL (8.4 MJ/l) and is cleared more rapidly than the 10% solution. Unlike hypertonic dextrose solutions, lipid emulsions are isotonic to plasma and can be infused through peripheral veins. The lipid emulsions

Table 5
Basic daily requirements for total parenteral nutrition

Nutrient	Amount
Water (kg body wt/day)	30–40ml
Amino acids (kg body wt/day)	
Medical patient	1.0g
Postoperative patient	2.0g
Hypercatabolic patient	3.0g
Minerals (for adults)	
Acetate/gluconate	90 mEq
Calcium	15 mEq
Chloride	130 mEq
Chromium	15 ug
Copper	1.5mg
Iodine	120 ug
Magnesium	20 mEq
Manganese	2 mg
Phosphorous	300 mg
Potassium	100 mEq
Selenium	100 ug
Sodium	100 mEq
Zinc	5 mg
Vitamins (for adults)	
Ascorbic acid	100 mg
Biotin	60 ug
Folic acid	400 ug
Niacin	40 mg
Riboflavin	3.6 mg
Thiamine	3 mg
Vitamin A	4000 IU
Vitamin D	400 IU
Vitamin E	150mg
Vitamin K	200 ug

are available in unit volumes from 50 to 500 mL and can be infused separately at a maximum rate of 50 mL/h or added to the dextrose-amino acid mixtures. Infused lipid is hydrolyzed by lipoprotein lipase, an enzyme present in the endothelial cells of blood vessels. Lipids that are not cleared from the circulatory system are at greater risk for being deposited in the lung and brain. Septic or severely stressed patients are impeded in their ability to clear intravenous lipid particles.

Electrolytes

Most electrolyte mixtures contain sodium, chloride, potassium, and magnesium; they also may contain calcium and phosphorous. The daily requirement for any specific electrolyte can be specified in the daily TPN orders. If no electrolyte requirements are specified, they are added to replace normal daily electrolyte losses.

Vitamins

Aqueous multivitamin preparations are added to the dextrose-amino acid mixtures. One unit vial of a standard multivitamin preparation provides the normal daily requirements for most vitamins.

Trace elements

Various trace element additives are available that contain chromium, copper, manganese, and zinc, but they do not contain iron and iodine. Table 5 illustrates daily requirements. Routine administration of iron is not recommended in critically ill patients because of pro-oxidant actions of iron.

Complications

Metabolic complications include hyperglycemia and hyperosmolality, which should be avoided by careful monitoring and by the administration of insulin. Hypoglycemia is precipitated by sudden discontinuance of constant concentrated dextrose infusion. Treatment consists of peripheral infusion of 5% or 10% dextrose for 24 hours before resuming central line feeding. Abnormalities of serum electrolytes and minerals should be detected by monitoring before symptoms and signs occur. Treatment involves appropriate modification of subsequent infusions or, if correction is required immediately, appropriate peripheral vein infusions. Vitamin and mineral deficiencies are most likely to occur during long-term TPN. Elevation of blood urea nitrogen occurs not infrequently during TPN and may result from hyperosmolar dehydration, which can be corrected by free water given as 5% dextrose by way of a peripheral vein. In adults, hyperammonemia is not a problem with currently available amino acid solutions. Liver dysfunction, evidenced by elevations of transaminases, bilirubin, and alkaline phosphatase, is common with the initiation of TPN, but these elevations are usually transitory and they are detected by regular monitoring. Delayed or persistent elevations may relate to the amino acid infusion, and protein delivery should be reduced. Painful hepatomegaly suggests fat accumulation, and the carbohydrate load should be reduced. Complications of parenteral nutrition include:

1. Metabolic complication—fluid overload, hypoglycemia, hyperglycemia, and hypercalcemia
2. Infectious complications—most often caused by staphylococcus epidermis and staphylococcus aureus
3. Metabolic bone disease—seen in patients receiving long term therapy. Patients may experience bone pain, bone fractures, and radiograph evidence of demineralization
4. Thrombosis and pulmonary embolous—radiologic evidence of subclavian vein thrombosis occurs commonly (25%–50% of patients), but clinical significant manifestations of pulmonary embolism are rare
5. Mechanical complications—during placement, the following complications can occur: pneumothorax, carotid or subclavian artery puncture, hemothorax, and thoracacio duct injury
6. Hepatobiliary complications—same patient may develop cholelithiasis, cholecystitis, elevated serum aminotransferase, and alkaline phosphatase.

Of nonmetabolic complications, pneumothorax and hematoma formation are the most common, but damage to other structures and air embolism have been reported. Proper placement of the catheter tip in the superior vena cava always must be confirmed by chest radiograph before infusion of TPN fluid. Complications that are related to central catheter placement should be less than 5%. Thromboembolism and catheter-related sepsis are the most common serious complications of TPN therapy. Common organisms include *Staphylococcus aureus, Candida* sp, *Klebsiella pneumoniae, Pseudomonas aeruginosa, S. albus,* and *Enterobacter* sp. Fever during TPN should be investigated and if no cause is found and the temperature remains elevated for greater than 24 to 48 hours, central catheter infusion should be stopped. Before the catheter is removed, blood for culture should be drawn directly from the central catheter and catheter infusion site. After removal, 2 to 3 inches of the catheter tip should be cut off with a sterile scalpel or scissors; placed in a dry, sterile culture tube; and sent for bacterial and fungal culture. Volume overload may occur when high, daily energy requirements necessitate large fluid volumes. Weight should be monitored daily; a gain of greater than 1 kg/d suggests volume overload and daily fluid delivery should be reduced.

Monitoring total parenteral nutrition support

The oral surgeon should make certain that a nutritional assessment is performed on his/her patient and that the nutritional support being delivered is safe and adequate to ensure normal healing. Adjustment of nutritional support during a long hospital stay in a severely traumatized patient is common because the clinical status of the patient may change. In certain patients it is important for the oral surgeon to monitor body weight, fluid intake, and fluid output daily. Once central parenteral nutrition (CPN) is started, serum electrolytes should be measured every 1 to 2 days until values are stable and then re-checked weekly. Serum glucose must be checked every 4 to 6 hours by finger stick until blood glucose concentrations are stable and then re-checked weekly. If lipid is being given, serum triglycerides should be measured.

Constant vigilance to the catheter and catheter site can help prevent infections. Gauze dressing should be changed every 48 to 72 hours or when contaminated or wet. Tubing that connects the parental solutions should be changed every 24 hours. When a single lumen catheter is used to deliver CPN, no other solution or medications, with the exception of compatible antibiotics, should be infused. When a triple lumen catheter is used the distal port should be reserved for the CPN.

Summary

Malnutrition in the oral and maxillofacial surgery surgical patient can have critical implications in the overall well-being and prognosis of the long-term, OMS hospitalized, ill patient. The OMS should be capable of assessing the patient's nutritional status and nutritional requirements and developing appropriate recommendations for proper nutritional management. Knowledge of the various modalities of nutritional support should be readily available to the OMS practitioner.

References

[1] Studley HO. Percentage of weight loss: a basic indicator of surgical risk in patients with chronic peptic ulcer. JAMA 1936;106:458–60.

[2] Erstad BL, Campbell DJ, Rollins CJ, et al. Albumin and prealbumin concentrations in patients receiving postoperative parenteral nutrition. Pharmacotherapy 1994;14:458–62.

[3] Carr CS, Ling KD, Boulos P, et al. Randomized trial of safety and efficacy of immediate postoperative enteral feeding in patients undergoing gastrointestinal resection. BMJ 1996;312:869–71.

[4] Hellin-Lopez J, Baena-Fustegueras JA, Schwartz-Riera S, et al. Usefulness of short-lived proteins as nutritional indicators in surgical patients. Clin Nutr 2002;21:119–25.

[5] Allison SP. Malnutrition, disease, and outcome. Nutrition 2000;16:590–3.

[6] Jagoe RT, Goodship TH, Gibson GJ. The influence of nutritional status on complications after operations for lung cancer. Ann Thorac Surg 2001;71:936–43.

[7] Huckleberry Y. Nutritional support and the surgical patient. Am J Health Syst Pharm 2004;61(7):671–82.

[8] Margenthaler JA, Herrmann VM. Nutrition. In: Doherty GM, Lowney JK, Mason JE, et al, editors. The Washington manual of surgery. 3rd edition. Philadelphia: Lippincott, Williams & Wilkins; 2002. p. 9–26.

[9] Demling RH, Desanti L. The stress response to injury and infection: role of nutritional support. Wounds 2000;12(1):3–14.

[10] Levy MM, Unger LD, Mullen JL. Nutritional considerations following trauma. In: Fonseca RJ, Walker RV, Betts NJ, editors. Oral and maxillofacial trauma. 2nd edition. Philadelphia: WB Saunders; 1997. p. 61–78.

[11] Poulin E. Prophylactic nutrition. Can J Surg 1991;34(6):555–9.

[12] Dabrowski GP, Rombeau JL. Practical nutritional management in the trauma intensive care unit. Surg Clin North Am 2000;3(1):11–5.

[13] Baker JP, Detsky AS, Wesson DE, et al. Nutritional assessment: a comparison of clinical judgment and objective measurements. N Engl J Med 1982;306:969–72.

[14] Katelaris PH, Bennett GB, Smith RC. Prediction of postoperative complications by clinical and nutritional assessment. Aust N Z J Surg 1986;56:743–7.

[15] Detsky AS, Baker JP, O'Rourke K, et al. Predicting

nutrition-associated complications for patients undergoing gastrointestinal surgery. JPEN J Parenter Enteral Nutr 1987;11:440–6.
[16] Gibbs J, Cull W, Henderson W, et al. Preoperative serum albumin level as a predictor of operative mortality and morbidity. Arch Surg 1999;134:36–42.
[17] Kudsk KA, Tolley EA, DeWitt RC, et al. Preoperative albumin and surgical site identify surgical risk for major postoperative complications. JPEN J Parenter Enteral Nutr 2003;27:1–9.
[18] Beck FK, Rosenthal TC. Prealbumin: a marker for nutritional evaluation. Am Fam Physician 2002;65(8): 1575–8.
[19] Stallings VA, Hark L. Nutritional assessment is medical practice. In: Morrison G, Hark L, editors. Medical nutrition and disease. Cambridge (MA): Blackwell Science; 1996. p. 3–31.
[20] Slone DS. Nutritional support of the critically ill and injured patient. Crit Care Clin 2004;20(1):135–57.
[21] Marino PL. Nutrition and energy requirements. In: Zinner SR, editor. The ICU book. Baltimore (MD): Williams & Wilkins; 1997. p. 721–36.
[22] Brandi LS, Bertolini R, Calafa M. Indirect calorimetry in critically ill patients: clinical applications and practical advice. Nutrition 1997;13(4):349–58.
[23] ASPEN. Board of Directors and the Clinical Guidelines Taskforce. Guidelines for the use of parenteral and enteral nutrition in adult and pediatric patients. JPEN J Parenter Enteral Nutr 2002;26(Suppl 1): 1SA–138SA.
[24] Prelack K, Sheridan RL. Micronutrient supplementation in the critically ill patient: strategies for clinical practice. J Trauma 2001;51:601–20.
[25] Erickson KL, Medina EA, Hubbard NE. Micronutrients and innate immunity. J Infect Dis 2000;182(Suppl 1): S5–10.
[26] Sauberlich HE. Human requirements and needs. Vitamin C status: methods and findings. Ann N Y Acad Sci 1975;258:438–50.
[27] Mueller DH, Burke F. Vitamin and mineral therapy. In: Morrison G, Hark L, editors. Medical nutrition and disease. Cambridge (MA): Blackwell Science; 1996. p. 46–66.
[28] Schorah CJ, Downing C, Piripitsi A, et al. Total vitamin C, ascorbic acid, and dehydroascorbic acid concentrations in plasma of critically ill patients. Am J Clin Nutr 1996;63(5):760–5.
[29] Russell RM. Vitamin and trace mineral deficiency and excess. In: Braunwald E, Facui AS, Kasper DL, editors. Harrison's principles of internal medicine. 15th edition (International edition, vol 1). New York: McGraw-Hill; 2001. p. 461–9.
[30] Howard L. Enteral and parenteral nutrition therapy. In: Braunwald E, Facui AS, Kasper DL, editors. Harrison's principles of internal medicine. 15th edition (International edition, vol 1). New York: McGraw-Hill; 2001. p. 470–8.
[31] Dwyer J. Nutritional requirement and dietary assessment. In: Braunwald E, Facui AS, Kasper DL, editors. Harrison's principles of internal medicine. 15th edition (International edition, vol 1). New York: McGraw-Hill; 2001. p. 451–5.
[32] Pietrzik K, Hesse CH, Zur Wiesch ES, et al. Urinary excretion of pantothenic acid as a measurement of nutritional requirements. Int J Vitam Nutr Res 1975; 45(2):153–62.
[33] Tao HG, Fox HM. Measurements of urinary pantothenic acid excretions of alcoholic patients. J Nutr Sci Vitaminol (Tokyo) 1976;22(4):333–7.
[34] Babior BM, Bunn HF. Megaloblastic anemia. In: Braunwald E, Facui AS, Kasper DL, et al, editors. Harrison's principles of internal medicine. 15th edition (International edition, vol 1). New York: McGraw-Hill; 2001. p. 674–80.
[35] Geerlings SE, Rommes JH, van Toorn DW, et al. Acute folate deficiency in a critically ill patient. Neth J Med 1997;51(1):36–8.
[36] Lawlor E, Watson A, Keogh JA. Folate deficiency in acute ill patients. Ir J Med Sci 1983;152(2):73–82.
[37] Bender DA. Optimum nutrition: thiamin, biotin and pantothenate. Proc Nutr Soc 1999;58(2):427–33.
[38] Mock DM, Henrich CL, Nadine Carnell N, et al. Indicators of marginal biotin deficiency and repletion in humans: validation of 3-hydroxyisovaleric acid excretion and a leucine challenge. Am J Clin Nutr 2002; 76(5):1061–8.
[39] Stephensen CB. Vitamin A, infection, and immune function. Annu Rev Nutr 2001;21:167–92.
[40] McCullough FS, Northrop-Clewes CA, Thurnham DI. The effect of vitamin A on epithelial integrity. Proc Nutr Soc 1999;58(2):289–93.
[41] Holick MF, Krane SM. Introduction to bone and mineral metabolism. In: Braunwald E, Facui AS, Kasper DL, et al, editors. Harrison's principles of internal medicine. 15th edition (International edition, vol 2). New York: McGraw-Hill; 2001. p. 2192–205.
[42] Takeda K, Shimada Y, Amano M, et al. Plasma lipid peroxides and alpha-tocopherol in critically ill patients. Crit Care Med 1984;12(11):957–9.
[43] Bertrand Y, Pincemail J, Hanique G, et al. Differences in tocopherol-lipid ratios in ARDS and non-ARDS patients. Intensive Care Med 1989;15(2):87–93.
[44] Shearer MJ. The roles of vitamins D and K in bone health and osteoporosis prevention. Proc Nutr Soc 1997;56(3):915–37.
[45] Booth SL. Skeletal functions of vitamin K-dependent proteins: not just for clotting anymore. Nutr Rev 1997; 55(7):282–4.
[46] Dardenne M. Zinc and immune function. Eur J Clin Nutr 2002;56(Suppl 3):S20–3.
[47] Darveau M, Denault AY, Blais N, et al. Bench-to-bedside review: iron metabolism in critically ill patients. Crit Care 2004;8(5):356–62.
[48] Adamson JW. Iron deficiency and other hypoproliferative anemias. In: Braunwald E, Facui AS, Kasper DL, et al, editors. Harrison's principles of internal medicine. 15th edition (International edition, vol 1). New York: McGraw-Hill; 2001. p. 660–6.

[49] Piagnerelli M, Vincent JL. Role of iron in anaemic critically ill patients: it's time to investigate!. Crit Care 2004;8(5):306–7.
[50] Hawker FH, Stewart PM, Snitch PJ. Effects of acute illness on selenium homeostasis. Crit Care Med 1990; 18:442–6.
[51] Angstwurm MW, Schottdorf J, Schopohl J, et al. Selenium replacement in patients with severe systemic inflammatory response syndrome improves clinical outcome. Crit Care Med 1999;27:1807–13.
[52] Heyland DK, Novak F, Drover JW, et al. Should immunonutrition become routine in critically ill patients? A systematic review of the evidence. JAMA 2001;286(8):944–53.
[53] Bastian L, Weimann A. Immunonutrition in patients after multiple trauma. Br J Nutr 2002;87(Suppl 1): S133–4.
[54] Sacks GS, Genton L, Kudsk KA. Controversy of immunonutrition for surgical critical-illness patients. Curr Opin Crit Care 2003;9(4):300–5.
[55] Alvarez W, Mobarhan S. Finding a place for immunonutrition. Nutr Rev 2003;61(6 Pt 1):214–8.
[56] Proceedings from Summit on Immune-Enhancing Enteral Therapy. San Diego, May 25–26, 2000. JPEN J Parenter Enteral Nutr 2001;25:S61–3.
[57] Klein S, Kinney J, Jeejeebhoy K, et al. Nutrition support in clinical practice: review of published data and recommendations for future research directions. National Institutes of Health, American Society for Parenteral and Enteral Nutrition, and American Society for Clinical Nutrition. JPEN J Parenter Enteral Nutr 1997;21(3):133–56.
[58] Gaddy MC, Max MH, Schwab CW, et al. Small bowel ischemia: a consequence of feeding jejunostomy? South Med J 1986;79(2):180–2.
[59] Moore EE, Jones TN. Benefits of immediate jejunostomy feeding after major abdominal trauma–a prospective, randomized study. J Trauma 1986;26(10): 874–81.
[60] Lewis SJ, Egger M, Sylvester PA, et al. Early enteral feeding versus "nil by mouth" after gastrointestinal surgery: systematic review and meta-anaylsis of controlled trials. BMJ 2001;323(7316):773–6.
[61] The Veterans Affairs Total Parenteral Nutrition Cooperative Study Group. Perioperative total parenteral nutrition in surgical patients. N Engl J Med 1991; 325(8):525–32.
[62] Stuart S, Stuart M, Unger LD. Enteral and parenteral nutrition support. In: Morrison G, Hark L, editors. Medical nutrition and disease. Cambridge (MA): Blackwell Science; 1996. p. 339–52.
[63] Falender LG, Leban SG, Williams FA. Postoperative nutritional support in oral and maxillofacial surgery. J Oral Maxillofac Surg 1987;45:324–30.
[64] Kudsk KA, Croce MA, Fabian TC, et al. Enteral versus parenteral feeding. Effects on septic morbidity after blunt and penetrating abdominal trauma. Ann Surg 1992;215(5):503–11 [discussion 511–13].
[65] Braunschweig CL, Levy P, Sheean PM, et al. Enteral compared with parenteral nutrition: a meta-analysis. Am J Clin Nutr 2001;74(4):534–42.
[66] Sigalet DL, Mackenzie SL, Hameed SM. Enteral nutrition and mucosal immunity: implications of feeding strategies in surgery and trauma. Can J Surg 2004;2(47):109–16.
[67] Braga M, Gianotti L, Gentilini O, et al. Early postoperative enteral nutrition improves gut oxygenation and reduces costs compared with total parenteral nutrition. Crit Care Med 2001;29(2):242–8.
[68] Marino PL. Enteral nutrition. In: Zinner SR, editor. The ICU book. Baltimore (MD): Williams & Wilkins; 1997. p. 737–53.
[69] Rees RG, Keohane PP, Grimble GK, et al. Elemental diet administered nasogastrically without starter regimens to patients with inflammatory bowel disease. JPEN J Parenter Enteral Nutr 1986;10(3):258–62.
[70] Marcuard SP, Stegall KS. Unclogging feeding tubes with pancreatic enzyme. JPEN J Parenter Enteral Nut 1990;14(2):198–200.
[71] Sriram K, Jayanthi V, Lakshmi RG, et al. Prophylactic locking of enteral feeding tubes with pancreatic enzymes. JPEN J Parenter Enteral 1997;21(6):353–6.
[72] Maloney JP, Ryan TA. Detection of aspiration in enterally fed patients: a requiem for bedside monitors of aspiration. JPEN J Parenter Enteral Nutr 2002; 26(6 Suppl):S34–41 [discussion S41–2].
[73] Ibanez J, Penafiel A, Marse P, et al. Incidence of gastroesophageal reflux and aspiration in mechanically ventilated patients using small-bore nasogastric tubes. JPEN J Parenter Enteral Nutr 2000;24(2):103–6.
[74] Strong RM, Condon SC, Solinger MR, et al. Equal aspiration rates from postpylorus and intragastric-placed small-bore nasoenteric feeding tubes: a randomized, prospective study. JPEN J Parenter Enteral Nutr 1992;16(1):59–63.
[75] Eisenberg P. An overview of diarrhea in the patient receiving enteral nutrition. Gastroenterol Nurs 2002; 25(3):95–104.

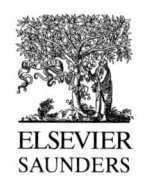

Index

Note: Page numbers of article titles are in **boldface** type.

A

Addiction, in surgical patients, 67–69

Age, patient, as risk factor for postoperative
  pulmonary complications, 83
  factor in wound healing, 109
  indications for preoperative testing based on, 5

Airway, upper, postoperative obstruction of,
  in patients with pulmonary disease, 86

Alcohol abuse, in surgical patients, 67–69

Ambulation, early, for postoperative risk reduction in
  patients with pulmonary disease, 91

American Society of Anesthesiologists (ASA),
  patient classification system, 2
    indications for preoperative testing based on,
    4–5

Amino acid solutions, in nutritional support of
  surgical patients, 126

Analgesia. *See* Pain management.

Anatomy, pediatric, perioperative considerations,
  35–37

Anesthesia, effect on respiration, in patients with
  pulmonary disease, 84–85
  general, for sedation in geriatric patients, 24–25
  local, for sedation in geriatric patients, 22

Anger, in oral surgical patients, 62–63

Antibiotics, prophylactic, for preoperative risk
  reduction in patients with pulmonary disease, 90
  preoperative, for subacute bacterial
  endocarditis, 41

Anticoagulant therapy, risks due to, in preoperative
  assessment of geriatric patients, 26–27

Anticonvulsants, fever due to, 76

Antimicrobials, fever due to, 76

Antithrombotic agents, for venous thromboembolism
  prophylaxis, 99–100

Anxiety, in oral surgical patients, 60–61
  preoperative, in pediatric patients, 42–43

Arthritis, preoperative assessment of, in geriatric
  patients, 31

ASA classification, indications for preoperative
  testing based on, 2–5

Aspiration, postoperative, in patients with pulmonary
  disease, 86

Aspirin, for venous thromboembolism prophylaxis, 99

Asthma, pediatric, as preoperative consideration, 40
  postoperative exacerbation of, 85–86

Atelectasis, postoperative, in patients with pulmonary
  disease, 86

Attention deficit disorders, in pediatric perioperative
  management, 43–44

Autologous blood donation, 15

B

Bacterial endocarditis, subacute, postoperative fever
  due to, 77–79
  preoperative antibiotic prophylaxis for, 41

Bioburden, or wound, interfering with wound
  healing, 108–109

Biomarkers, of nutritional status, 116–117

Blood components, perioperative therapy with, 14–15

Blood products, perioperative usage of, **12–16**
  anticipation of usage, 12–13
  autologous usage, 15
  blood component therapy, 14–15
  complications of usage, 15
  end parameters of volume resuscitation,
  15–16
  indications for blood therapy, 14
  volume resuscitation, 13–14

Bronchospasm, postoperative, in patients with
  pulmonary disease, 88

C

Calcium, in perioperative fluid and electrolyte management, 11–12

Caloric requirements, in nutritional support of surgical patients, 118

Caloric studies, to assess nutritional status, 117–118

Cancer, venous thromboembolism prophylaxis in patients with, 101

Cardiovascular disease, preoperative assessment of, in geriatric patients, 25–27
in pediatric patients, 40–41
mitral valve prolapse, 41
murmurs, 41
subacute bacterial endocarditis, antibiotic prophylaxis for, 41

Cardiovascular medications, fever due to, 76
risks due to, in preoperative assessment of geriatric patients, 26–27

Cerebrovascular disease, preoperative assessment of, in geriatric patients, 27–28

Chronic obstructive pulmonary disease (COPD), as risk factor for postoperative pulmonary complications, 82
postoperative exacerbation of, 85–86

Cognitive evaluation, and informed consent in geriatric patients, 21

Components, blood, perioperative therapy with, 14–15

Compression devices, intermittent pneumatic, for venous thromboembolism prophylaxis, 99

Compression stockings, graduated, for venous thromboembolism prophylaxis, 99

Cryoprecipitate, indications for perioperative therapy with, 15

Cystic fibrosis, pediatric, as preoperative consideration, 40

D

Deep vein thrombosis, prophylaxis of, for postoperative risk reduction in patients with pulmonary disease, 90–91

Delirium, postoperative, in geriatric patients, 31

Dementia, preoperative assessment of, in geriatric patients, 31

Depression, in oral surgical patients, 61–62

Dextrose solutions, in nutritional support of surgical patients, 126

Diabetes mellitus, preoperative assessment of, in geriatric patients, 29–31

Diagnostic testing, preoperative, 1–6

Direct thrombin inhibitors, for venous thromboembolism prophylaxis, 100

Drug addiction, in surgical patients, 67–69

Drug dosages, for pediatric patients, 45

Drug fevers, 76

E

Edema, postobstructive pulmonary, in patients with pulmonary disease, 86–87

Education, patient, for preoperative risk reduction in patients with pulmonary disease, 90

Electrolytes. *See also* Fluid and electrolyte management.
in nutritional support of surgical patients, 127

Embolism, pulmonary, postoperative, in patients with pulmonary disease, 87–88

Emergency care, of pediatric patients, legal considerations, 45–46

Emotions, impact on oral surgical patients, 59–60

Endocarditis, subacute bacterial, postoperative fever due to, 77–79
preoperative antibiotic prophylaxis for, 41

Endocrine disorders, preoperative assessment of, in geriatric patients, 29–31

Energy requirements, in nutritional support of surgical patients, 118

Enteral nutrition, in perioperative care, 123–124
products for, 124–125
protocol for, 125

Evaluation. *See* Preoperative evaluation.

F

Factor VIII, indications for perioperative therapy with, 15

Factor Xa inhibitors, for venous thromboembolism prophylaxis, 100

Fasting, preoperative, guidelines for pediatric patients, 44–45

Fat-soluble vitamins, in nutritional support of surgical patients, 121

Fever, postsurgical, **73–79**
 causes of, 75
 chemical mediators of, 73–74
 definition of, 73
 drug fevers, 76
 due to malignant hyperthermia, 77–79
 due to subacute bacterial endocarditis, 77–79
 fever-reducing agents, 74–75
 treatment, 79
 within 24 to 72 hours after surgery, 76–77
 within the first 24 hours, 75–76
 workup of, 79

Fluid and electrolyte management, perioperative, **7–12**
   calcium, 11–12
   in pediatric patients, 44
   magnesium, 12
   normal exchange of, 7–9
   phosphate, 12
   sodium, 9–11

Fresh frozen plasma, indications for perioperative therapy with, 15

G

General anesthesia, in geriatric patients, 24–25

Geriatric patients, perioperative care for, **19–34**
   general medical history, 19–22
     cognitive evaluation and informed consent, 21
     medications, 21
     nutrition and fluid electrolytes, 19–20
     social history, 20–21
   risk assessment of comorbid systemic disease, 25–32
     arthritis, 31
     cardiovascular disease, 25–27
     cerebrovascular and neurologic disease, 27–28
     dementia and postoperative delirium, 31–32
     endocrine disorders, 29–31
     respiratory disease, 28–29
   sedation strategies for, 22–25
     general anesthesia, 24–25
     inhalation, with nitrous oxide, 22
     intravenous, 23–24
     local anesthesia, 22
     oral, 22–23

Graduated compression stockings, for venous thromboembolism prophylaxis, 99

H

Healing, of wounds, **107–113**

Health status, as risk factor for postoperative pulmonary complications, 83

Hemodynamic considerations postoperative, 56

Hemorrhage, acute, classification of, 14

Heparins, for venous thromboembolism prophylaxis, 100

Hip fracture surgery, venous thromboembolism prophylaxis in patients undergoing, 101

History, patient, in presurgical nutritional assessment, 116
 indications for preoperative testing based on, 5

Hypercalcemia, perioperative management, 12

Hyperkalemia, perioperative management, 11–12

Hypermagnesemia, perioperative management, 12

Hypernatremia, perioperative management, 10–11

Hyperphosphatemia, perioperative management, 12

Hypertension, preoperative assessment of, in geriatric patients, 26
 pulmonary, as risk factor for postoperative pulmonary complications, 83

Hyperthermia, malignant, postoperative fever due to, 77–79

Hypokalemia, perioperative management, 10–11

Hypomagnesemia, perioperative management, 12

Hyponatremia, perioperative management, 9–10

Hypophosphatemia, perioperative management, 12

Hypoxemia, postoperative, in patients with pulmonary disease, 86

I

Immunocompetence, measures of, to assess nutritional status, 117

Immunonutrition, in nutritional support of surgical patients, 122–123

Infections, pediatric respiratory, as preoperative consideration, 40

Informed consent, in geriatric patients, cognitive evaluation and, 21
 in pediatric patients, 45

Inhalation sedation, in geriatric patients, 22

Intravenous sedation, in geriatric patients, 23–24

L

Laboratory testing, preoperative, recommended guidelines for, **1–6**
    ASA patient classification, 2
    indications for, 4–5
    surgical classification, 3
    universal algorithm for, 3

Legal considerations, in pediatric care, 45–46
    emergency care, 45–46
    informed consent, 45

Lipid emulsions, in nutritional support of surgical patients, 126–127

Local anesthesia, for sedation in geriatric patients, 22

Lung disease, as risk factor for postoperative pulmonary complications, 82–83

Lung expansion maneuvers, for postoperative risk reduction in patients with pulmonary disease, 90

M

Macrominerals, in nutritional support of surgical patients, 121–122

Magnesium, in perioperative fluid and electrolyte management, 12

Malignancy, venous thromboembolism prophylaxis in patients with, 101

Malignant hyperthermia, postoperative fever due to, 77–79

Malingering, in perioperative patients, 67

Medications, as factor in wound healing, 111
    in perioperative risk assessment of geriatric patients, 21–22

Microminerals, in nutritional support of surgical patients, 121–122

Micronutirents, in nutritional support of surgical patients, 118–119

Mitral valve prolapse, pediatric, as perioperative consideration, 41

Murmurs, heart, pediatric, as perioperative consideration, 41

Muscular dystrophy, pediatric, as perioperative consideration, 42

N

Nausea, and vomiting, postoperative management of, 55–56

Neurologic disease, preoperative assessment of, in geriatric patients, 27–28

Neuromuscular disorders, pediatric, as perioperative consideration, 41–42

Nitrogen balance studies, to assess nutritional status, 117–118

Nitrous oxide, inhalation sedation with in geriatric patients, 22

Nonsteroidal anti-inflammatory drugs (NSAIDs), for postoperative pain, 53–54

Nutrition, in perioperative care, **115–130**
    assessment of, in surgical patients, 115–116
    biomarkers of nutritional status, 116–117
    caloric and energy requirement, 118
    caloric and nitrogen balance studies, 117–118
    enteral nutrition, 123–124
        products for, 124–125
        protocol for, 125
    fat-soluble vitamins, 121
    immunocompetence, measures of, 117
    immunonutrition, 122–123
    macrominerals, 121–122
    microminerals, 122
    micronutrients, 118–119
    parenteral nutrition, 125–128
        amino acid solutions, 126
        complications, 127–128
        dextrose solutions, 126
        electrolytes, 127
        lipid emulsions, 126–127
        monitoring, 128
        trace elements, 127
        vitamins, 127
    protein requirements, 118
    soluble vitamins, 119–121
    timing, 123
    in perioperative risk assessment of geriatric patients, 19–20
    poor, as factor in wound healing, 110

O

Obesity, as risk factor for postoperative pulmonary complications, 83

Obstructive sleep apnea, as risk factor for postoperative pulmonary complications, 82

Opioids, for postoperative pain, 53

Oral sedation, in geriatric patients, 22–23

Over-the-counter drugs, in perioperative risk assessment of geriatric patients, 21

Oxygenation, postoperative, 50–51

Oxygenation, tissue, poor, as factor in wound healing, 109–110

P

Pain management, medications for, in perioperative risk assessment of geriatric patients, 21–22
    postoperative, 51–54
        NSAIDs, 53–54
        opioids, 53
        pre-emptive analgesia, 52–53

Parental presence, in the operating room, 43

Parenteral nutrition, total, in perioperative care, 125–128
    amino acid solutions, 126
    complications, 127–128
    dextrose solutions, 126
    electrolytes, 127
    lipid emulsions, 126–127
    monitoring, 128
    trace elements, 127
    vitamins, 127

Pediatric patients, perioperative considerations in, **35–47**
    anatomy and physiology, 35–37
    drug doses in, 45
    evaluation of, 38–39
    fluid and electrolyte management in, 44
    legal considerations in, 45–46
    preoperative fasting guidelines in, 44–45
    psychologic considerations in, 42–44
    system-specific conditions in, 39–42
        cardiovascular, 40–41
        neuromuscular, 41–42
        respiratory, 39–40

Perfusion, tissue, poor, as factor in wound healing, 109–110

Perioperative care, 1–130
    blood products, **12–16**
        anticipation of usage, 12–13
        autologous usage, 15
        blood component therapy, 14–15
        complications of usage, 15
        end parameters of volume resuscitation, 15–16
        indications for blood therapy, 14
        volume resuscitation, 13–14
    fever, postsurgical, **73–79**
        chemical mediators of, 73–74
        definition of, 73
        drug fevers, 76
        due to malignant hyperthermia, 77–79
        due to subacute bacterial endocarditis, 77–79
        fever-reducing agents, 74–75
        treatment, 79
        within 24 to 72 hours after surgery, 76–77
        within the first 24 hours, 75–76
        workup of, 79
    fluid and electrolytes, **7–12**
        calcium, 11–12
        magnesium, 12
        normal exchange of, 7–9
        phosphate, 12
        sodium, 9–11
    in geriatric patients, **19–34**
        general medical history, 19–22
        risk assessment of comorbid systemic disease, 25–32
        sedation strategies for, 22–25
    in pediatric patients, **35–47**
        anatomy and physiology, 35–37
        drug doses in, 45
        evaluation of, 38–39
        fluid and electrolyte management in, 44
        legal considerations in, 45–46
        preoperative fasting guidelines in, 44–45
        psychologic considerations in, 42–44
        system-specific conditions in, 39–42
            cardiovascular, 40–41
            neuromuscular, 41–42
            respiratory, 39–40
    in pulmonary disease patients, **81–94**
        perioperative complications in, 83–88
        preoperative assessment of risk, 81–83
        risk reduction strategies, 88–91
    laboratory and diagnostic testing, preoperative, **1–6**
        ASA patient classification, 2
        indications for, 4–5
        recommended guidelines, 2–5
        surgical classification, 3
        universal algorithm for, 3
    nutritional aspects of, **115–130**
        assessment of, in surgical patients, 115–116
        biomarkers of nutritional status, 116–117
        caloric and energy requirement, 118
        caloric and nitrogen balance studies, 117–118
        enteral nutrition, 123–124
            products for, 124–125
            protocol for, 125
        fat-soluble vitamins, 121
        immunocompetence, measures of, 117
        immunonutrition, 122–123
        macrominerals, 121–122

microminerals, 122
microminutrients, 118–119
parenteral nutrition, 125–128
    amino acid solutions, 126
    complications, 127–128
    dextrose solutions, 126
    electrolytes, 127
    lipid emulsions, 126–127
    monitoring, 128
    trace elements, 127
    vitamins, 127
protein requirements, 118
soluble vitamins, 119–121
timing, 123
postoperative care, **49–58**
    hemodynamic considerations, 56
    nausea and vomiting, 55–56
    pain management, 51–54
    temperature, 54
    urine output, 54–55
    ventilation and oxygenation, 50–51
    wound care, 56–57
psychologic considerations, **59–72**
    anger, 62–63
    anxiety, 60–61
    depression, 61–62
    factors complicating the surgical event, 67–69
        addicted patients, 67–69
        malingering and secondary gain, 67
    impact of emotions on oral surgery patients, 59–60
    pretreatment considerations, 64
    somatoform disorders or somatic complaints, 63–64
    techniques for patient preparation, 65–67
venous thromboembolism, **95–105**
    epidemiology, 95–96
    incidence of in oral surgery patients, 96
    pathogenesis and natural history, 95
    prevention of, 98–103
        duration of prophylaxis, 102
        in different clinical situations, 100–102
        mechanical methods, 99
        pharmacologic agents, 99–100
        rationale for, 100
        strategies for improvement of in hospitals, 102
        vena cava interruption, 99
    risk factors for, 96–98
wound healing and, **107–113**

Phosphate, in perioperative fluid and electrolyte management, 12
    perioperative fluid and electrolyte management, 12

Physical examination, in presurgical nutritional assessment, 116
    indications for preoperative testing based on findings from, 5

Physiology, pediatric, perioperative considerations, 35–37

Plasma expanders, perioperative usage of, 14

Plasma, fresh frozen, indications for perioperative therapy with, 15

Platelets, indications for perioperative therapy with, 15

Pleural effusion, postoperative, in patients with pulmonary disease, 87

Pneumatic compression devices, intermittent, for venous thromboembolism prophylaxis, 99

Pneumonia, postoperative, in patients with pulmonary disease, 87

Postoperative care, of oral and maxillofacial surgery patients, **49–58**
    hemodynamic considerations, 56
    nausea and vomiting, 55–56
    pain management, 51–54
    temperature, 54
    urine output, 54–55
    ventilation and oxygenation, 50–51
    wound care, 56–57

Postoperative fever. *See* Fever, postsurgical.

Potassium, perioperative fluid and electrolyte management, 10–11

Pre-emptive analgesia, for postoperative pain, 52–53

Pregnancy, venous thromboembolism prophylaxis in, 101–102

Preoperative evaluation, in pediatric patients, 38–39
    laboratory and diagnostic testing in, **1–6**

Preoperative laboratory testing, **1–6**
    recommended guidelines, 2–5
        ASA patient classification, 2
        indications for, 4–5
        surgical classification, 3
        universal algorithm for, 3

Prophylaxis, of venous thromboembolism, 98–103

Protein requirements, in nutritional support of surgical patients, 118

Psychologic considerations, in pediatric perioperative management, 42–44
   attention deficit disorders, 43–44
   parental presence in the operating room, 43
   preoperative anxiety, 42–43
in perioperative care, **59–72**
   anger, 62–63
   anxiety, 60–61
   depression, 61–62
   factors complicating the surgical event, 67–69
      addicted patients, 67–69
      malingering and secondary gain, 67
   impact of emotions on oral surgery patients, 59–60
   pretreatment considerations, 64
   somatoform disorders or somatic complaints, 63–64
   techniques for patient preparation, 65–67

Pulmonary disease, perioperative care in patients with, **81–94**
   perioperative complications in, 83–88
      changes in pulmonary interstitium, 84
      effect of anesthesia on respiration, 84–85
      pathophysiology, 83
      postoperative complications, 85–88
      ventilation, 83–84
   preoperative assessment of risk, 81–83
      pulmonary function testing, 81–82
      risk factors for postoperative complications, 82–83
   risk reduction strategies, 88–91
      intraoperative strategies, 90
      postoperative strategies, 90–91
      preoperative preparation, 88–90

Pulmonary edema, postobstructive, in patients with pulmonary disease, 86–87

Pulmonary embolism, postoperative, in patients with pulmonary disease, 87

Pulmonary function testing, 81–82

Pulmonary hypertension, as risk factor for postoperative pulmonary complications, 83

Pulmonary interstitium, postoperative changes of, in patients with pulmonary disease, 84

Pyrogens, 73–74

R

Radiation injury, as factor in wound healing, 110–111

Red blood cells, indications for perioperative therapy with, 15

Respiratory disease, preoperative assessment of,
   in geriatric patients, 28–29
   in pediatric patients, 39–40
      asthma, 40
      cystic fibrosis, 40
      infections, 39–40

S

Scars, principles of wound care, 112–113

Secondary gain, in perioperative patients, 67

Sedation, in geriatric patients, perioperative strategies for, 22–25
   general anesthesia, 24–25
   inhalation, with nitrous oxide, 22
   intravenous, 23–24
   local anesthesia, 22
   oral, 22–23

Sleep apnea, obstructive, as risk factor for postoperative pulmonary complications, 82

Smoking, risk factor for postoperative pulmonary complications, 82
   risks due to, in preoperative assessment of geriatric patients, 29

Smoking cessation, preoperative, for risk reduction in patients with pulmonary disease, 88–89

Social history, in perioperative risk assessment of geriatric patients, 20–21

Sodium, in perioperative fluid and electrolyte management, 9–11

Soluble vitamins, in nutritional support of surgical patients, 119–121

Somatic complaints, in oral surgical patients, 63–64

Somatoform disorders, in oral surgical patients, 63–64

Subacute bacterial endocarditis, postoperative fever due to, 77–79
   preoperative antibiotic prophylaxis for, 41

Substance abuse, in surgical patients, 67–69

Surgical classification system, indications for preoperative testing based on, 3–5

T

Temperature, in postoperative care, 54

Thromboembolic complications. *See also* Venous thromboembolism.
   risks due to, in preoperative assessment of geriatric patients, 29

Thyroid disease, preoperative assessment of, in geriatric patients, 30–31

Tissue perfusion and oxygenation, poor, as factor in wound healing, 109–110

Total parenteral nutrition. *See* Parenteral nutrition, total.

Trace elements, in nutritional support of surgical patients, 127

Tracheal laceration and perforation, postoperative, in patients with pulmonary disease, 88

Trauma, venous thromboembolism prophylaxis in patients with, 101

U

Upper airway obstruction, postoperative, in patients with pulmonary disease, 86

Urine output, postoperative, 54–55

V

Vena cava interruption, for venous thromboembolism prophylaxis, 99

Venous thromboembolism, **95–105**
　epidemiology, 95–96
　incidence of in oral surgery patients, 96
　pathogenesis and natural history, 95
　preoperative risk reduction in patients with pulmonary disease, 89–90
　prevention of, 98–103
　　duration of prophylaxis, 102
　　in different clinical situations, 100–102
　　mechanical methods, 99
　　pharmacologic agents, 99–100
　　rationale for, 100
　　strategies for improvement of in hospitals, 102
　　vena cava interruption, 99
　risk factors for, 96–98

Ventilation, postoperative, 50–51
　complications of, in patients with pulmonary disease, 83–84

Vitamin K antagonist, for venous thromboembolism prophylaxis, 100

Vitamins, in nutritional support of surgical patients, fat-soluble, 121
　soluble, 119–121

Volume resuscitation, perioperative blood product usage for, 13–16
　autologous blood usage, 15
　blood component therapy, 14–15
　complications, 15
　end parameters of, 15–16
　indications for, 14

Vomiting, nausea and, postoperative management of, 55–56

W

Wound healing, **107–113**
　factors interfering with, age, 109
　　concomitant disease, 110
　　medications, 111
　　poor nutrition, 110
　　poor tissue perfusion and oxygenation, 109–110
　　radiation injury, 110–111
　　wound bioburden, 108–109
　how wounds heal, 107–108
　postoperative management, 56–57
　principles of wound care, 111–113
　　full-thickness wounds, 112
　　partial-thickness wounds, 112
　　scars, 112–113
　　wound closure, 111–112

Changing Your Address?

Make sure your subscription changes too! When you notify us of your new address, you can help make our job easier by including an exact copy of your Clinics label number with your old address (see illustration below.) This number identifies you to our computer system and will speed the processing of your address change. Please be sure this label number accompanies your old address and your corrected address—you can send an old Clinics label with your number on it or just copy it exactly and send it to the address listed below.

We appreciate your help in our attempt to give you continuous coverage. Thank you.

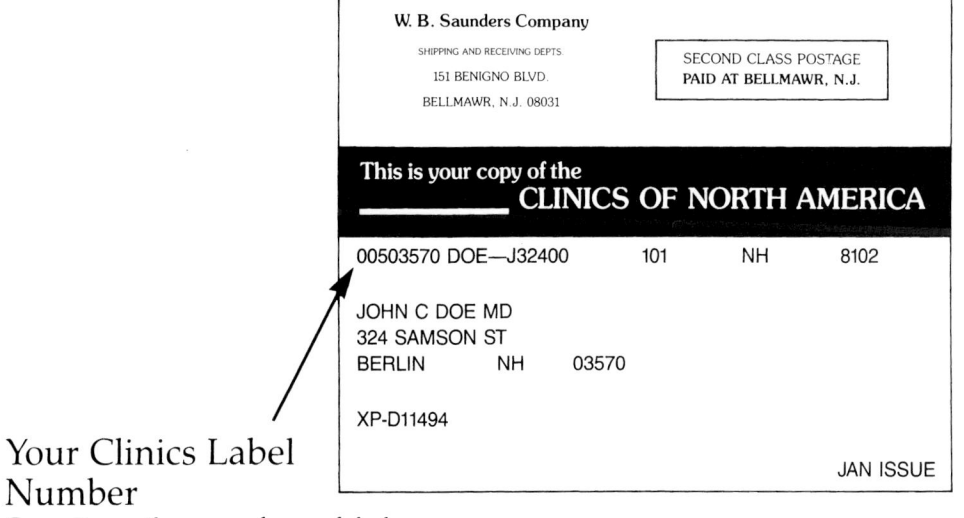

```
W. B. Saunders Company
SHIPPING AND RECEIVING DEPTS.
151 BENIGNO BLVD.
BELLMAWR, N.J. 08031

SECOND CLASS POSTAGE
PAID AT BELLMAWR, N.J.

This is your copy of the
_____ CLINICS OF NORTH AMERICA

00503570 DOE—J32400      101      NH      8102

JOHN C DOE MD
324 SAMSON ST
BERLIN      NH      03570

XP-D11494

JAN ISSUE
```

Your Clinics Label Number
Copy it exactly or send your label along with your address to:
W.B. Saunders Company, Customer Service
Orlando, FL 32887-4800
Call Toll Free 1-800-654-2452

Please allow four to six weeks for delivery of new subscriptions and for processing address changes.